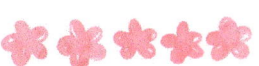

Honored Grief

Carolina -Ayala- Velasquez

Honored Grief/ Carolina M-G Ayala---
1st ed
ISBN 979-8-9855006-6-0

Printed in the United States Of America

Disclaimer and Trauma Warning

Grief can be a heavy topic that can bring up many emotions and thoughts. More than the author shared experiences, that can sometimes activate emotions or trigger things. People will share personal experiences, with no filters.

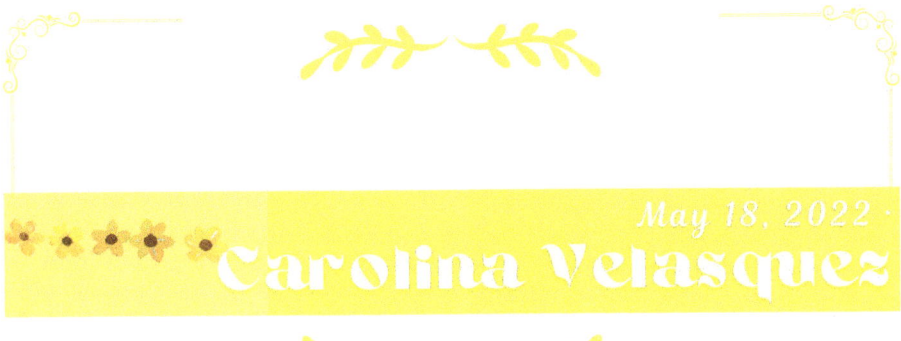
I think there is something very powerful about showing up as you are; about being unpolished, unrehearsed, and real. No one can tell your story like you can.

We all have stories to tell. I think honesty creates opportunity for release and healing; and it also creates the space to make genuine connections. I thank you for being a part of making my dream a reality by supporting me on this author journey.

I am not just living a child-hood dream or life-long dream. I am living many dream come trues every time I get to create a book. I release with its imperfections because I want you and everyone to know— you can create a book and live your dream without being "perfect", as long as it is good enough for you.

I am a life-long learner. I will continue to learn and grow and teach. I will continue to share my whole self, in hopes to inspire others to do the same.

I want to see us all win. I want to help us all "make it." I could never do anything "alone", I am never alone.

I have so much happiness seeing my husband's cousins name on the cover of this book. She is an amazing artist of many talents and I am so grateful that two of her paintings are the cover. I am so thankful to have her as the illustrator.

Any way that I can support my family and friends, is helping me create a life I once only dreamed of.

Sharing grief and gratitude with the world, in this way- is helping me live in my life's purpose.

This book is not perfect. It is imperfectly perfect and it is yet again, just one of many to come.

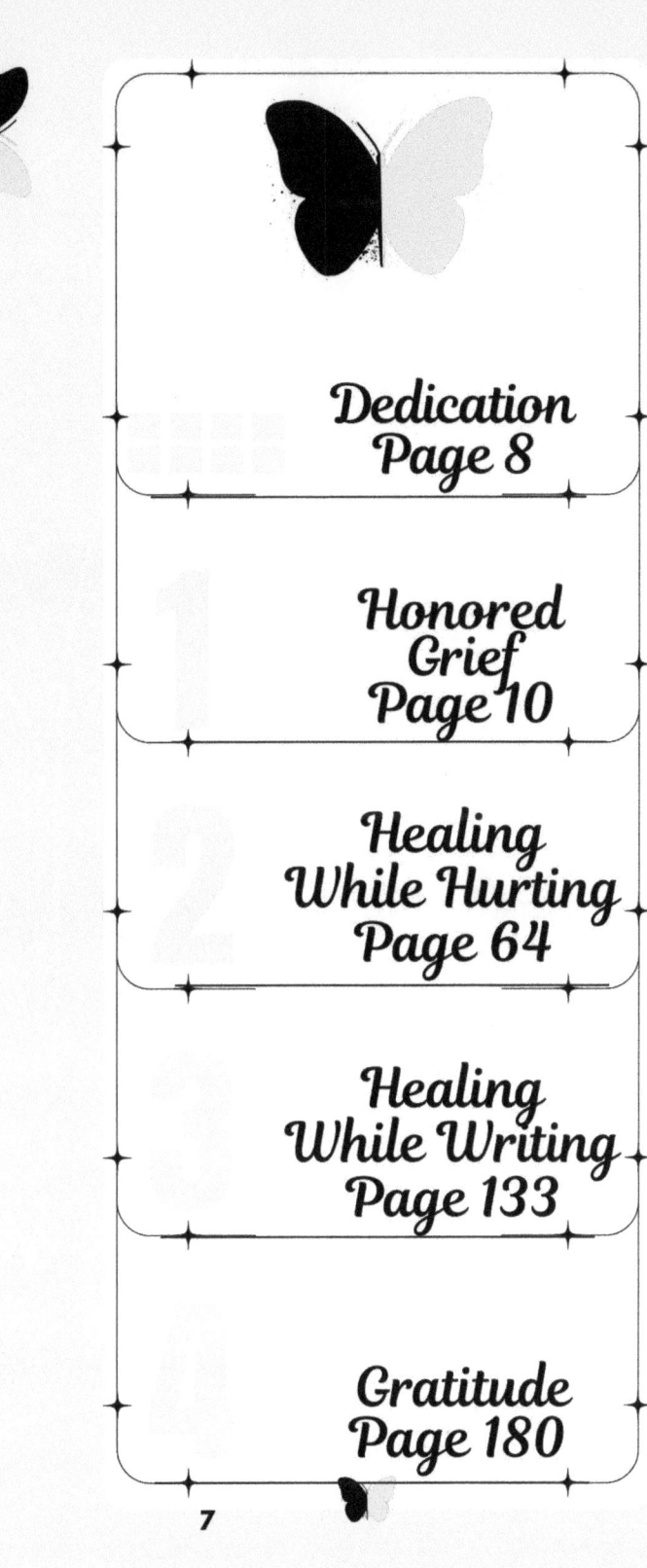

CONTENTS

Dedicated to my loved
one's who have
transitioned.
To my loved ones who are
grieving.

And, in honor of:
Juan Ramon Ayala

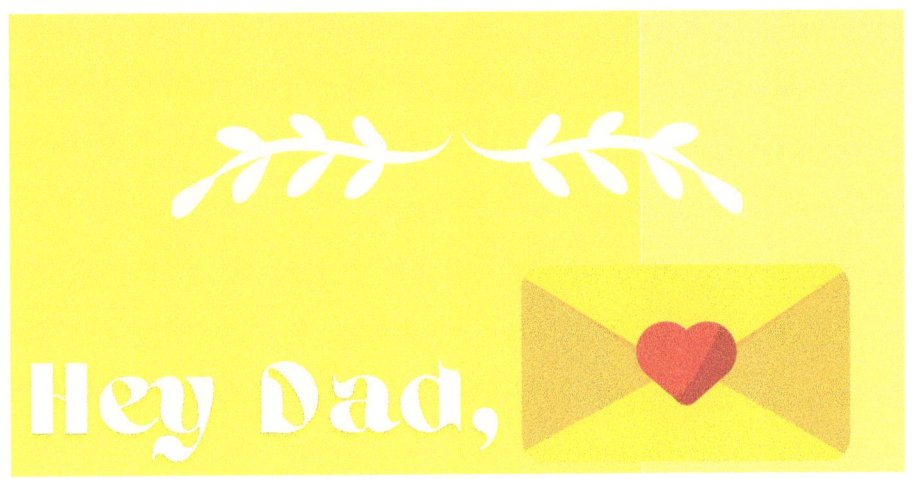

Hey Dad,

It is me again. Making a new book, in honor of your 10-year anniversary of your transition this month of January 2024.

The message and feeling continues that I am doing this to honor and celebrate you and my journey when it comes to grief and healing. I hope this book helps keep memories alive, love alive, hope alive and healing happening.

I started all of this so long ago. I shared and learned that what I was going through could also help others relate, help others share their stories and honor their truths, to let others know they are not alone and that in feeling our feelings-there is space for healing.
I hope this reminds and shows anyone that your voice and words and feelings matter.
You are your super-power.

Thank you, dad, for continuing to work through me, by inspiring me to do for you which in return helps me live in my dream and purpose and not just for myself but to include others I love along the way as a community.

Chapter

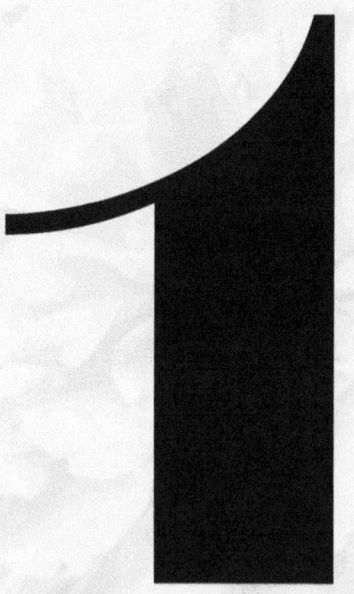

1

Honored Grief

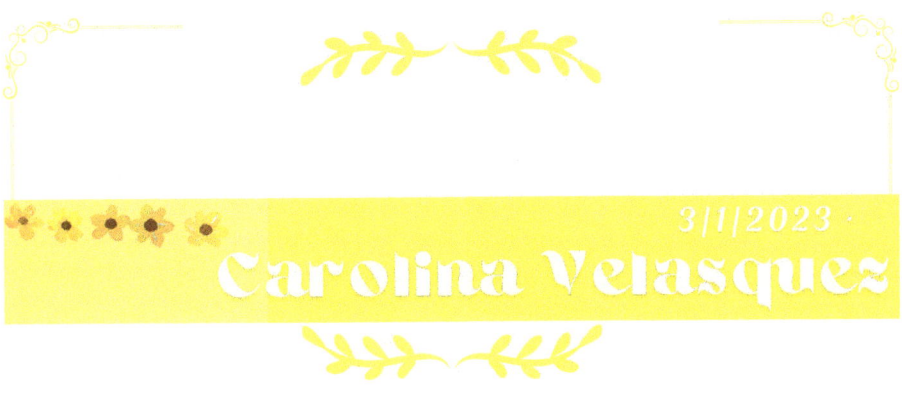

Carolina Velasquez

Writing has been healing for me.
Feeling my pain has been my medicine instead of a band aid.

Honored grief is a compilation of "healing while hurting" and "healing while writing." It is also its own book with pieces added in that don't exist in the previous books made.

In December 2023 I created a grief and gratitude card deck for myself, inspired by both books + more added from my journey of podcasts I was guest on & workshops I lead and spaces I spoke in. When I created that deck, I decided I wanted to create a book +card deck together for 2024.

This combination book would be "honored grief" because both healing while hurting and healing while writing are about how I honor my grief. How I honor my journey through reflection, sharing and creating.
And this is how "honored grief" was born.

How do you honor your grief?

I have learned some of the ways I honor my grief is by allowing what is real to be. Reflecting on my feelings, thoughts, and experiences. I am a documenter in many ways (pictures, diary, timestamps...)
Many times, I come up with questions based on what is going on, it is how I make sense and dive deeper.

I turn them into journal prompts, I share my words with "the world" and sometimes I hear reflections back from people. That is a ripple effect. That, to me- is healing in many forms.

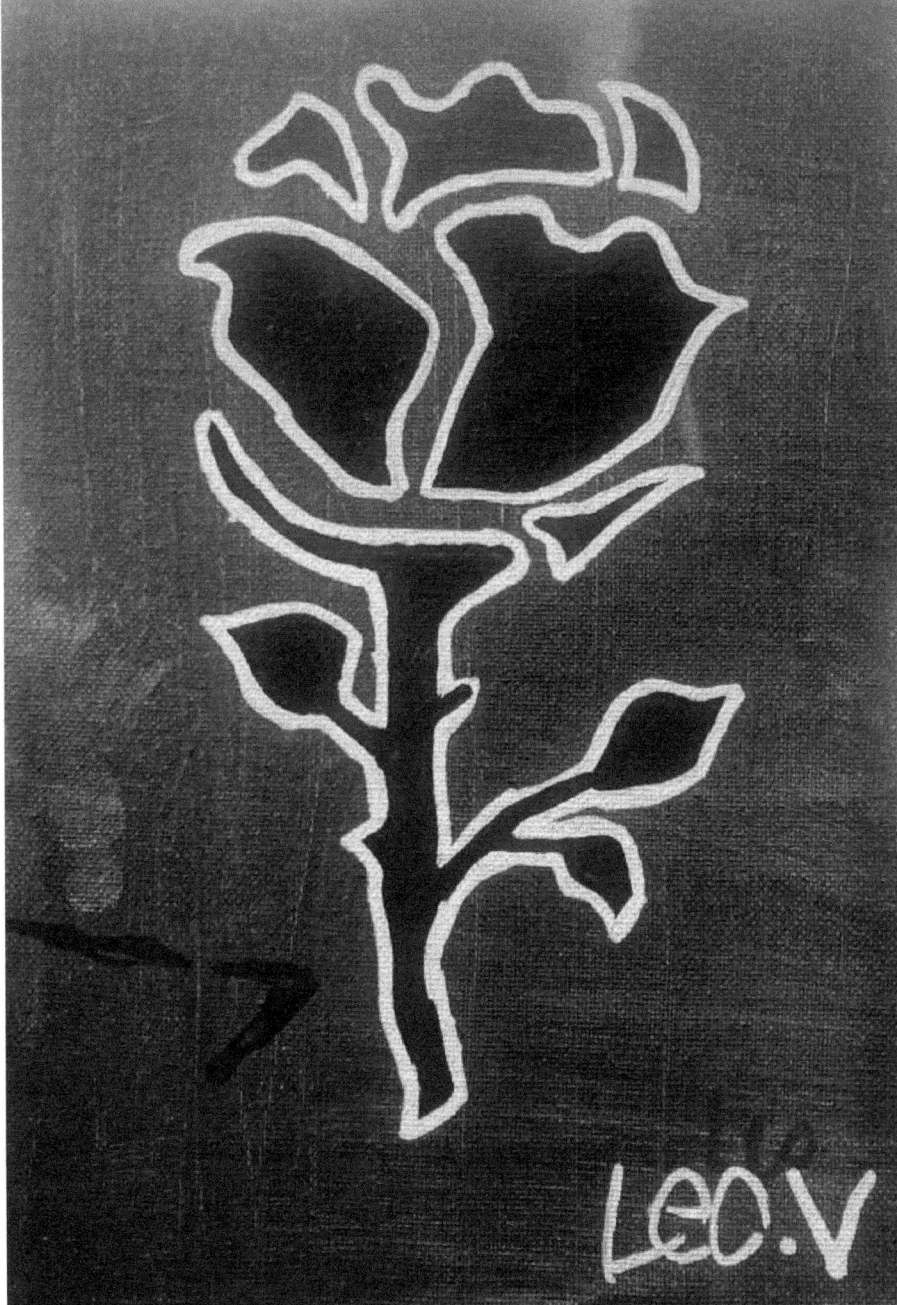

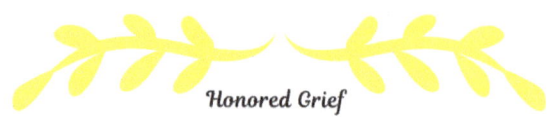

Today is January 14, 2024. The day I said my rough draft would be "done."

I was talking to my husband asking if he would be willing or wanting to be included in the book. We talked about how this could look. He asked me why it mattered to me. Then it came to me- to offer the idea and invitation out to those I know---aka fb and ig.

So I Shared:

I am working on a book (I wrote 90% last year) but want to add pieces in. Which means it can't be 100 without it.

"Honored Grief"

Is about the ways we honor our grief. Our ancestors. Our loved ones. Our hearts. Our journey.

It is a book that has a mix of "healing while hurting" + "healing while writing"

My hope is it can be on its own or paired with a card deck that is also a mix of both worlds (reflections/prompts) for those who like to journal or be inspired for poetry or reflection.

This month is my dad's 10-year anniversary.
Of course, I want to honor him.

****A thought just came to me, which is where my ask/invitation comes in---
for anyone it speaks to....

I would you like to be included in this book?
-you can write a message for my dad or my family. It can be a memory you'd like to share or a thought or prayer or quote, whatever. An intention.

or---/and--- you could answer a question (whatever resonates) and I can enter it in the book.... (I can use your name or nickname or no name- whatever you feel called)

- How do you honor those who have transitioned?
- What lessons has grief taught you
- What does your grief want you to know?
- When it comes to grief, what are you grateful for?
- What is grief? what does it mean to grieve? how does it feel in your body and show in your actions?
- What does it feel/look like to heal while on the grief journey?

There cannot be a wrong or right answer. Only a real one. Part of my purpose on this earth, the reason I write and share---a reason I became a self-published author----
is because I want to help others in feeling safe/proud/able to take the leap in sharing their truths.

I share, in hopes it supports anyone else to do the same.
Part of my path is to lift others up, to helps others be seen and held and heard.
To use whatever "platform" I have- and share voices, share messages.

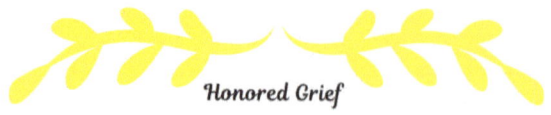

If you'd like to dedicate your words or writing to anyone/several names---please feel free to share that as well and I would love to add that in as well.

I have learned, when we share our stories- you never know who or how it may help someone. Even if that someone is you.

Right away I was blown away with personal messages and comments on my post. I feel honored.

Here is where I will share, those who asked to be shared in this way. Here, is how we grieve and heal-in community and individually.

Consider these next pages both a dedication and a "thank you"

This is how we, honor grief:
(Our grief, our healing, our truth, our journey, our ancestors, our stories, our experiences, our hearts...)

> I have healed and walked through my own grief with words from Lena. How she has led me through this journey is powerful, magical, soothing and it just feels right. I will always indebted to you for all the ways your words have touched my soul... And may you Always write and share. God bless you and your family
> - Kathy Munoz

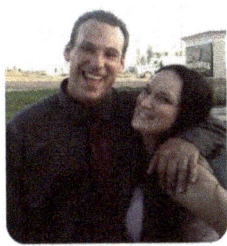

SOME ONE, SOME WHERE, KNOWS SOMETHING! WHERE ARE YOU CORY?!

> Thank you for being the father figure and protector I needed growing up.
> Miss you forever, love you for always. -Amy Perry

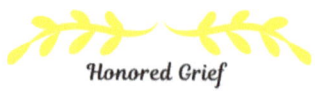

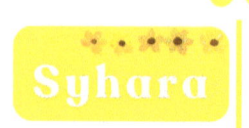

Syhara

Grief is weird to me. One day you can look at a photo of your person and smile, and the next day or moment you see the same photo you're crying, missing them, wishing they were here, wishing for one more chance to say something. Grief is like a wave, it comes and goes and sometimes it comes in heavy.

When my friend Maria passed away I couldn't even process it. It's been two years and I still haven't processed it. I believe that's because when she passed away I was so far away, I couldn't even make it for the funeral so to me it still isn't real. but I see her photos and instantly I am reminded when I try to reach out to her. The tears just come unexpectedly.

When Martha passed away I felt the same way, it isn't real because I'm not there to see it, to feel it.. I come across her photos and videos and I am filled with so much love and so much sadness because I know my next visit won't be the same.
That's just from the top of my head
When Raleigh, chats dad passed away, he didn't really react. It scared me at first, why aren't you in tears?

Why aren't you grieving the same way I've grieved or seen others grieve? Grief is different for everyone. Chats dad died when he was on vacation in another country. Chats way of grieving is different from mine.

He sits in silence and gives a quiet space for his feelings and emotions for his loss. His has his alter where he honors him.

I know that I need to start really processing Maria & Martha's passing. And that starts with honoring them in special ways. I feel closest to Maria when I'm in the car, that's when I think of her the most!

Whenever we were together, we were always dancing to cumbias or bachata, anything in Spanish really. I always feel like she's right there with me whenever I'm dancing. I feel closest to Martha when I'm praying. Her faith always touched me.

Whenever I would talk to her she always prayed with me, and told me that I'm smart, beautiful. And when I'm cooking anything Mexican lol. My tattoos always remind me that are here with me

> I needed to talk about it a little bit, open that up,
> To healing and processing.
> Love you thank you for this.

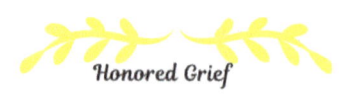

Anna Eddings

*My Tribute To My
Friend And Brother
Juan Ayala*

Remember clear as if it were today, when and where I met Juan. I remember his big smile and those pearly whites! I'm smiling just thinking of him . It was a sunday and I was visiting a church in san jose with my late husband Richard.

I see Richard's face just light up, and he yells out, "Juan!!!, I look up and see Juan walking towards us and the 2 embrace
I sincerely have to say, I had never seen Richard light up with anyone like he did with Juan that day. He introduced us and talked about what a good guy and good friend Juan was. It was sweet. Juan looked back at Richard with the same administration. I kid you not, it was a genuine moment between the 2 men.

After that, Juan and I became fast friends. Juan threw a surprise party for Richard, gathering a few old friends from back in the day that Richard hadn't seen in years. I remember it was so cool listening to these friends tell stories and laughing. We sure did laugh a lot. That was also a great day because I met Juan's daughter Carolina. ..

Juan was a very generous person. He was kind and thoughtful and had a quiet strength about him.

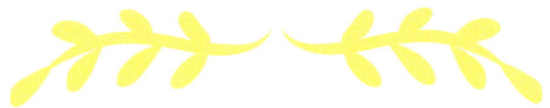

After Richard's passing, Juan was a pillar of support for me. He really did see me through some sad and lonely times, not just for me but also my family.
I have so many great memories in the short time that we were able to spend together.

Reflecting on our friendship, I truly am blessed to have cross paths with Juan, and I am truly grateful for our time together.
And I'm grateful to have been given this platform and the chance to share those memories.

I want to end with a quote about my dear friend Juan.

"When someone you love becomes a memory, the memory becomes a treasure."
Always in my heart Juan and I'll see you again my friend. LOVE ANA.

Thank you for allowing me to be a part of your book. It was like visiting with Juan while reliving the memories.

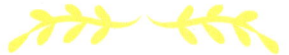

Rachel Brewer

Grief has taught me to cherish my memories more. Take more pictures, make more posts, anything to make the memory stick. But also, to spend more time with my loved ones. Even little moments like grocery shopping or organizing a room.

Our time is limited and never guaranteed so we must treat every moment as if the next one won't come. I lost my mother in 2016 and my step mother in 2022. I have lost countless family members over the years and now take every opportunity to see who I still have whenever I can.

I dearly miss Carol Van Diggelen and Barbara Brewer but their memories live on in me and my stories forever. After my mom passed, I tried to suppress memories, they hurt too much. But after I lost my step mother, I realized the memories are all I have. I've learned to be comfortable telling the stories and showing the pictures.

They can live on through me. As I get older I realize that it's ok to hurt and miss them, that will never stop. But I can smile and laugh and know they are looking down on me here and that they aren't in pain. I heal a little more every time I talk about them. And now I know I can help others to navigate their grief as well.

You can put whatever you want in the book, and my name is fine. If it helps you help another grieving then it's worth it.

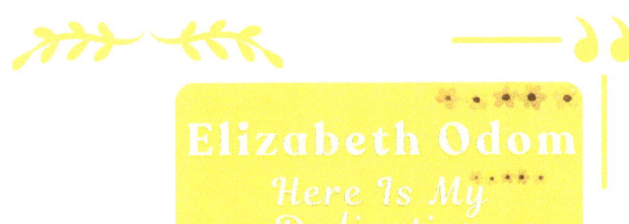

Grief is consuming, painful, real, and never ending. It changes your perspective on life and daily experiences. I have learned to embrace it and feel it. No one can take the place of the person you lost. You just need to allow yourself to feel. Know that it's okay to be happy, lost in love and content. welcome the pain just as much as you do love.

Memories are precious, find a way to keep them near you and allow yourself to remember the good times, you deserve it. I still have moments where I want to talk to my mom, tell her things, share, and just hold her hand. It's heart wrenching to realize I can't. Then again, I thank God she isn't suffering anymore.

All Saints suffered somehow, went through trials and tribulations before they left this world… it brings me peace to know there is some kind of end to the pain. With knowing God is there waiting to welcome our love ones a place to rest. Until we meet again.

It's ok if this doesn't make it in the book, I just want to share my thoughts, feelings and experiences with grief. I know you understand💛 rest well.

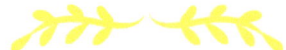 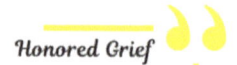
Darlene Low

I got the book you sent me you had me crying and I don't cry much but thank you. I love you and Loui's known you all your life, remember? I was the one that took your mother to the hospital and I was in the delivery room. When you came, Poppin out I guess I was there for a lot of the name things I was there when you first start School when you graduated And for holidays. Making your Easter basket when i made Paula and Rico's.

When you got married. For most of the important things. And when your dad would get you on a weekend to spend time with you or take you to a movie. Yea that was me. I love you Lena and so proud of the person you are. I love you more than my words would express.

You know me my words may not come out perfect but you know what I am trying to say. Stay strong and go for everything you want in life. Life is too short just be the person you are and you will accomplish much. I will always love you.

My words may of came out kinda wrong but you know what I am trying to say. I don't know if I'm doing this right but I'm talking to the phone and it's writing what I have to say, there's a lot I want to say but like you said you're not a therapist you're not a psychologist you're just a wonderful person that I am very proud of.

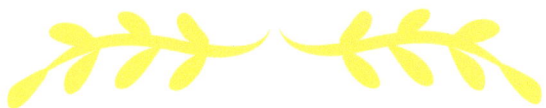

In your book you left spaces so people can write their feelings their comments or whatever I didn't want to mess up my book so I wrote it on paper now I'm telling the phone.

Anyway first of all I really like this book. Talking about your loved ones who have passed, I said damn I could say something about most of them, I know most of them- for you to mention Louie was so thoughtful, Lani and I can't express how much it meant. he knew you all your life but he was also your Dad's friend for many years before you were born, now you're right to help in grieving.

What is grieving they say- I have not taken the time to grieve, is there a time limit? is there a certain way to grieve? I know the way you feel that your loved one is gone the pain, the emptiness don't go away. they say time will make you feel better it don't you just learn to accept it.

They say your loved one is always with you. me I grew up believing in spirit so I know Louie is around here, we dream of him and listen to the message he is giving us he is always in our thoughts. my grandkids and I talk about him all the time. we get together and listen to oldies and talk about remember when Grandpa did this or that.

When he took them to their games ball games or just dropping them off at school and picking them up. remember this or remember that, he is always in our memories -he will never be forgotten.

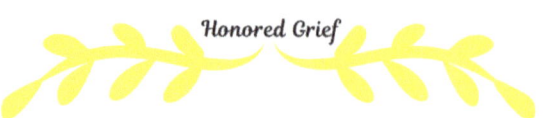

There is more to this that I want to write to you or to express my feelings but I'll do it a little at a time. this is what I wrote down so far but there is more than I want to express. I love you Lena and I always will and as I always say so proud of you. Lani and I can't express how much it meant to us for you to mention Louie.

Okay, this is the next part. You are lucky you got to be with your dad until the end. I couldn't be with Loui because of the corona. He was able to talk to us with that zoom. It was hard for him to talk because he had that oxygen. And his body was shutting down.

One of the last things I told him was-If he was tired, he said Yeah, I told him not to worry about us. We will be okay. I asked him if he wanted to go with his mother and sisters and family, he said. Yeah, I told him to just rest. Lay down and rest. And they're waiting for him with open arms. I told him it was okay, don't worry about us. All the time I wanted to say, stay strong. Come home, we want you home, we love you.

But I didn't want to put that stress on him Knowing that couldn't happen, he couldn't operate without that machine, his body was shutting down. I couldn't be that selfish, letting him go at least he wouldn't be in any more pain. Suffering by himself.

That's why I picked the poem that is in back of his card. I also know it would be selfish of me to let all the pain and heartache take over me cause I don't think i

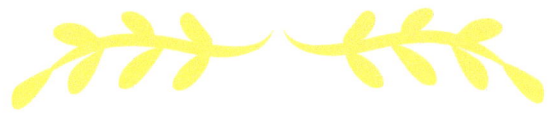

could really handle it. Than what would these kids do? they would be devastated. Maybe I am looking too far in the future.

But Louie is gone and we can't bring him back. We can just keep his memory.

With us forever.

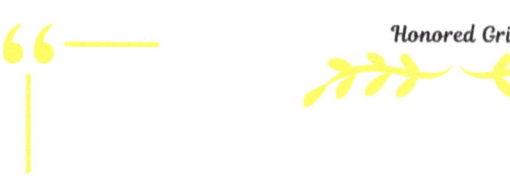

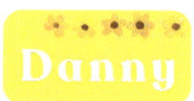

Folks it's said that the reason teenagers are assholes is due to the dangers of inbreeding.

You see, it's much easier to avoid children with four legs or no eyes if you avoid breeding amongst your immediate kin. Theoretically, teens develop a deep distain bordering on disgust towards their parents in order to insure they both leave the tribe to seek out new mates, and that they drive their parents nuts enough to want them out of the igloo asap.

Those families in which this behavior was common survived the tens of thousands of years as hunter gatherers and those who did not became mutated, slow minded sabretooth tiger meals.

Fast forward to. Modern society. Today's teens still exhibit this eye-rolling condescension towards their elders and inevitably fly the coop for more genetically advantageous peeps. All except maybe various royals and a few folks in the Appalachia. But I digress. I am no different than the average American guy.

As a kid, my parents were flawless. Always right, never made mistakes and certainly smarter than everyone else's. Teen years set in and I became more knowledgeable, morally correct, socially adept and certainly better looking than the troglodytes who held the keys to the prison they held me in for their own sick amusement.

Then I moved out.

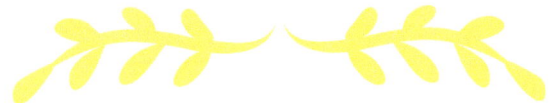

Things quickly changed and I began to make mistakes not unlike my firmer owners had. My flaws mirrored theirs, my humanness showed and it begun to be clear that all the foolish advice they attempted to bestow on my genius teenaged self was actually right. I no longer saw them as flawless, nor village idiots.

I saw them for the first time as people. Funny, loving, mistake-making, best intentioned people struggling to do their best with what they had, and doing a pretty damned good job of it.

I saw traights in myself that were directly and unavoidably like my father's, and my mothers. Although some I hated, I learned to recognize them and navigate the cultural, behavioral, and genetic quirks just as they had.

I lost both of them no more than 10 years ago now. I miss them both so deeply it feels as if a part of myself has died and will never be found. The pain and sadness don't hit me as frequently as they used to but the heart heavy tears still roll at the sound of a voice similar to my mom's, or when i say something my dad used to say.

The smell of a box of buttons That was my mom's has begun to fade. I'd open it frequently just to remember. My dad's old tube of hair grease still smells the same. Mom's voice is still clear but small memories are slowly fading. Like grandma's Danish cookie tin of crayons, one day it will lose all its smell and become just a tin of old, paperless, dirty crayons.

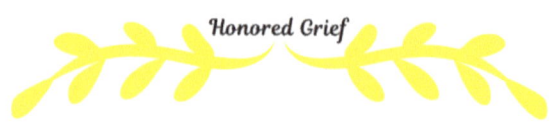

I keep things of theirs. Moms sewing machine, dads guns, nanas old dresser, and most importantly, my moms stained glass lamps. She was a really amazing artist. I used to wish I'd let her know that when she was alive. I regretted not doing so until my therapist asked why I don't do it now. I guess I kinda felt stupid writing a letter to no one but I trusted his advice and did so.

I let her know what an amazing mom she was and how a admired her creativity. That it inspired me and made me who I am today. I also forgave her for things she felt guilt towards.

Things I dont think she even understood. Things that people do. Because we're people and we all make mistakes.
I love you MA and Pops.

———**"**

Chantal Giordano

Honoring people who passed away is just thinking about them. Some things grief taught me was you should really talk nicer to people because you never know when they are going to go. I try not to think about the person for awhile because all you do is get sad when you think of someone who passed.

When my mom passed away, I told myself that she was just at my sister's house (which she was, cremated) When my sister Denise passed away- I just told myself she was at someone's house and I just can't see her right now----I guess that means I avoid dealing with it, even now.

Everyone who passed away makes me sad when I think about them. When I pass, I want people to honor me by not being sad. Why wait until I am dead, give me roses now.

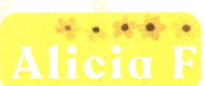

Alicia F

When I first got word that my mom passed away, I rushed home and as I walked in her room before they took her body away, the first thing I saw was a calendar with a scripture that said "FEAR NOT" in big bold letters. Even though I knew the journey ahead of me would be hard, God's message to me was fear not. I then felt a ray of peace that through my grief, I would be OK

Maria Paula Ahumada

And its ok to cry sometimes because you purposefully made yourself sad.

And its ok to cry because you miss her in the smallest way
And its ok to cry because your heart feels heavy
Its also ok to cry because you're scared

And its ok to not stop crying for a long time
You also get to take breaks whenever you want and for as long as you want
This is your time to heal and to love and to love stronger than ever before.

"As I am sitting here thinking about what to write about grief, I keep thinking about this poem I wrote a few years ago.

I would like to use this; I am also sending you love to you and your family as your dad's 10 years anniversary comes up.

Love you friend and thank you for allowing me to be a part of your writing".

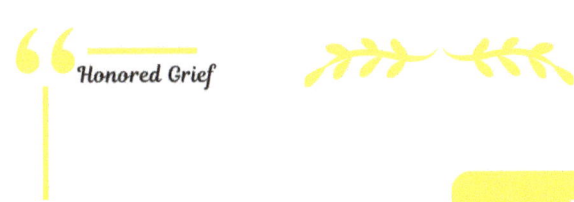

Edgardo Velasquez -Mora

To me, grief is what you feel when you lose someone or something important to you.

I honor loved ones who passed by praying to them before I leave the house, I try to hold conversation with their spirit in my alone time. The hardest part about losing someone, is that someone being my mom. To not be able to see her or talk to her again.

What I have done to support my grief is I let myself feel when I need to feel. Staying in prayer and remembering helps me cope. I try not to focus on things like what could I have done, I try not to focus on things I can't change.

I try to honor her by focusing on what is in front of me and what I can change. I kept myself busy mentally and physically like with coaching youth soccer, working, soaking in other people's moments who know me and relate to losing loved ones and feeling grief.

Something that stood out that someone said was "you have to let them be, to let them rest in peace" and sometimes I really feel that, I never want my mom to have to worry even in the afterlife-I want her to know I will be ok and continue to do better and be better than my past self.

Doing things that make me happy make me feel like I

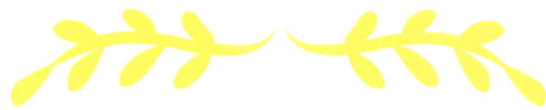

am healing. I know what I do for myself gives me a better chance at a better headspace and physical self. This journey is not easy.

A message to my mom is just how grateful I am for all of the moments that we came across. The challenging moments and how we grew better.

The life lessons. I still think she was gone too soon and I know I can't dwell on that and that one day we will be together again. I know she was proud and will be proud when we meet again.

Thankful for her love.

—"

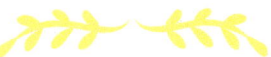
Jasmin Ancheta

Embracing Santosha: Navigating the Layers of Motherhood and Grief

I was about 6 months pregnant and sitting on the couch catching up on my favorite reality TV show "90 Day Fiancé" waiting for my husband to come home from work. I hear a knock at the door and outside the window, I see my husband struggling to get up the stairs with the rest of the baby haul.

I opened the door and everything came tumbling into our home, a stroller, car seat, baby clothes, shoes, accessories, baby toys, bassinet, you name it. Our small living room was suddenly filled with baby stuff and it dawned on me at that moment that our lives as we knew it was going to change.

I sat there staring at everything blankly while my husband was so excited to share all the things we got for the baby. He noticed I wasn't as enthusiastic as he was and asked me what was wrong I continued to stare blankly at all the baby stuff surrounding us and this feeling of sadness washed over me and I couldn't help but cry.

35

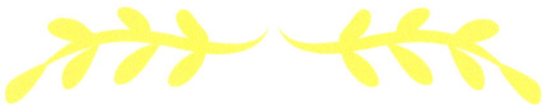

I remember telling him, "Our lives are going to change drastically and while my heart is filled with gratitude for all the things we have for our baby, I am still sad that our lives as we know it are going to be so different in just a couple of months."

Perhaps there was a part of me that was not done enjoying the life we built together, just us two and our two fur babies. The life we built finally felt simple. We are both in stable careers, traveling as we pleased, we just got married and it felt like we finally got a grip on this adulting thing.

To see our lives changing rapidly felt like I was losing control of what finally felt simple and grounding. Mom's around me prepared me for all the sleepless nights, the diaper blowouts, and the breastfeeding tips, but no one prepared me for the grieving I would feel as I transition into motherhood.

I wonder if anyone else has gone through this? Am I the only one? Does naming what I'm feeling out loud make me a bad mom? I suddenly have more questions than answers.

A few weeks after I had my meltdown, I remember watching a movie and there was a scene where they talked about the stages of grief. Denial, anger, bargaining, depression, and acceptance.

It was at that moment that I realized that what I was experiencing was the stages of grief. To be honest, when I thought about grief, I thought it meant grieving

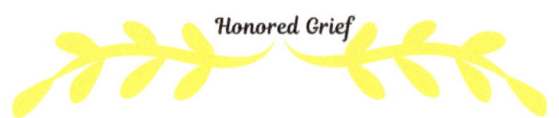

I lost friend, family, or pet that passed on to the other side. I never thought I could grieve a life I once knew. Hearing about the stages of grief helped me put a name to what I had been feeling for months. I had been in denial of our lives changing up until my husband brought home the baby gifts,

I was in sadness when I realized some things, we were able to do so easily might not be so easy with a baby, I was bargaining my energy by trying to do the most in my business as I usually do, but that bargaining quickly lead to burnout. Not only was my life changing, but I was changing and I had no idea who I was becoming.

When I delved into the stages of grief, I noticed that the last stage was acceptance. Drawing from the yogic philosophy santosha (contentment or accepting things as they are), I realized I could accept the ebbs and flows of my pregnancy or I could continue to resist it.

From that moment forward I made a conscious effort to allow what is to be, to find gratitude for my journey, and ground in my inner knowing that God has perfectly curated my life as it needs to be.

This lesson of grief taught me the coexistence of joy and sadness, gratitude, and grief. Life's complexities are not confined to black and white; they unfold in layers. Embracing Santosha became my anchor, allowing me to navigate the intricate tapestry of emotions and experiences with acceptance.

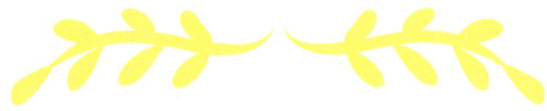

If my story resonated with you at all, I would love to connect, my Instagram handle is @healing.soulution I also have a podcast "Unfolding" that can be found on Apple Music and Spotify.

I hope I have the honor of connecting with you

"

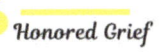

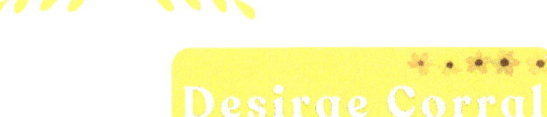

1O years ago, the world lost a wonderful man who could brighten up a whole room with his HUGE SMILE. Juan, thank you for always being so nice and smiling that bright smile at me. You are truly missed and forever in our hearts.

Lena, Thank you for sharing your dad with the world. I know he is so proud of you and all that you have accomplished. Your dad may be your angel now, but you were his angel here on earth.

Edgardo, I know Juan is so proud of you for the man you have become. You are taking such great care of his daughter and his grandchildren. He's rooting you on from Heaven.

Angel, Iris and Leo, Boy, did your grandpa LOVE you three so much! You guys made him so happy. I know you didn't get a lot of time with him, but I hope you all know how much he loved you.

Athena, I know you didn't get to meet your grandpa, but I know he would have loved you so much. Just know he sends you his love from Heaven. May God continue to comfort and wrap his arms around you all.

Those we love don't go away. They walk beside us every day. Unseen,unheard but always near, so loved, so missed.

Thomas J Edwards

Dearest Lena, thank you for inviting me to join you in this truly sacred moment.

As I contemplated on what I could possibly add that would be meaningful, thinking about our dads and wondering if they're out there conspiring for this moment to happen, this is what arrived. It's not something I've shared with very many people, definitely not in a very long time.

Within days of my dad's passing, as my mom and I began to slowly clean out his belongings, she had found a folded piece of paper. In his handwriting, in blue ballpoint ink, there was a quote. Just the quote. No context, no clues as to why he thought it important enough to write it down.

"There is a silent strength within each soul, and that strength is multiplied for those who remember that they do not walk their path alone."

Bernadette

We felt in our hearts in that moment that that was meant for us. Maybe for me.

She let me keep that paper, and I still have it with me today, over a decade now since he left.
I know my dad wanted me to share it with you.

Side note: I have no idea who Thomas J. Edwards is, but his name was written on the paper. I'm unsure who

40

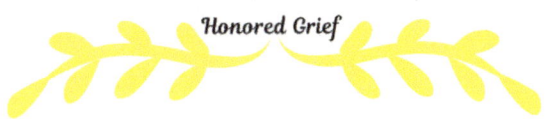

the original author of this quote is, in spite of a pretty robust effort to find it.

With love, Bernardo's Daughter, Bernadette

—„

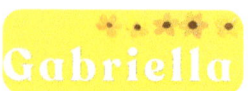

How do you honor those who have transitioned? Well for me, I listen to music it's my therapy .

- What lessons has grief taught you? Our physical life span is limited, but if we value our time alive it's priceless.

- What does grief want me to know? Hmm, I would like to say it wants me to know all the love you hold within for one another is forever, the pain of missing someone you love hurts but knowing the love is forever it's a beautiful blessing.

- When it comes to grief, what are you grateful for? Time. The time I had with my loved one and and the time it takes to heal is endless.

- What is grief? What does it mean to grieve? How does it feel in the body and your actions? My grief is pain my grief is tears. My grief is also a many sleepless nights wishing I could rewind time. Sometimes it's even breathtaking. It's the only thing in this world that someone can "help" me with.

- What does it feel/ look like to heal on your grief journey? It's one of the most painful journeys I've been on in my lifetime. when I first lost my loved one, I lost myself I lost sight of life. physically I gained weight and I didn't want to be around

42

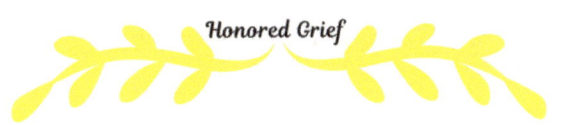

family. I felt broken. Then I met this beautiful soul who helped me get into and with myself who understood death and taught me how to grieve properly. I don't wanna sound cliché, but Lena you showed me that grief has no limit and that it's okay to hurt. It's hard to understand it that way because I was sad of being sad and I wasn't sure if it was just me. I didn't feel alone.

My message to Juan Ayala, I know I never met you physically but your daughter let's the whole world know who you are, through her eyes, feelings, words and the love she has for you. It's beautiful. I know your proud.
May your soul forever rest in peace. Love Gabriella.

— "

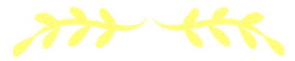
What did grief teach me?
Grief taught me how to love.
In the thick of grieving and depression I was sleep deprived but always exhausted, not wanting to eat and not getting out of bed, not even sure if I was breathing from moment to moment, I have learned my nervous system was going into freeze and fawn.

Because I saw grief as overwhelming, foreign, and dangerous. A tsunami crashing over me and taking me out to the sea. At the mercy of every swell of grief hoping it would not swallow me whole. I could either fight these waves of intense emotion or I could float or even ride these waves. As a descendant of the people of the ocean, I too could navigate these waters and wayfind my way back home.

Grief taught me to question: why is receiving affirming care so hard to receive? The systems were designed that way. While I also wished someone would come to feed me, rock me to sleep, witness my loss and anger, grief showed me this world will place barriers in my mind and physical and financial restraints on my community so that communal care freely given is inaccessible.

Grief led me down the rabbit hole of decolonization shedding light on areas I never knew needed healing from religion to parenting to my relationship with money/capitalism, the land, and traditional expectati-

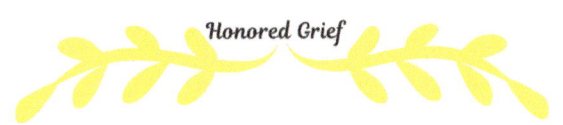

ons of leadership. Grief exposed me and challenged me to better. I broke up with religious and spiritual beliefs that made me believe I was anything less than divine, sacred, and precious and in turn demanded of the church that they be the vessel of love that unmarried itself from American politics.

I had to unlearn adultism and punishment to raise up fiercely loving, wise and liberated children. I discovered that fear managed my money so I had to heal my inner child and speak to her heart that I am always deserving and always provided for. I literally put to rest my addiction to hustle culture; this nervous system will be regulated by all means necessary.

I had no connection, no reverence for the land and nature so I planted seeds. And as a good mother would do, I nurtured my plants, learned what would help my plant family thrive and in turn they honor my efforts and provide the medicine. We take care of each other.

I was reminded that Spirit/God/Universe/the ancestors do not call the qualified; She qualifies the called. Grief has taught me I was born for this certain time for certain people in this certain place. Grief, through decolonizing, taught me that I am everything I need.

Grief has taught me to fiercely love myself and birthed a new life of unshakeable peace. My story is the medicine. My life is the curriculum. I am the fire. I am light. I am love. There is no time but now.

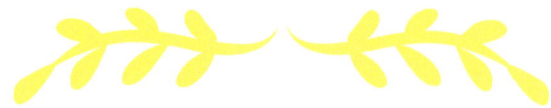

My ancestors walk with me. I am abundantly provided for and divinely sourced. All that is for me flows to me with ease. God ain't done with me yet because I woke up today.

And God isn't done with you yet. Because you are here reading these words. May you find yourself, your joy and your purpose as you navigate your grief and heal towards your own liberation.

This is dedicated to:

Roddy Calonsag who always taught me to laugh even when shit hits the fan. I know you are always cheering me on.
Kim Arbis Vazquez who embodied love and kindness always.
Tita Bec Jiz de Ortega who loved life and served with love to all around her. A mother to all.
Lolo Rudolph Calonsag who showed me that ministry was beyond the 4 walls of church, to put God first, eat good food, take the good and leave the bad, and speak only when it was necessary.

Alfie Gonzalez for working with me from another dimension and teaching me about my power.
Congressman John Lewis for showing me the best of Christians are those who seek justice, that ordinary people can do extraordinary things, and that good trouble is always necessary in a colonial world.

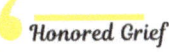

When my mother passed, I found myself between two grievances. One was the loss of my mother and the other was the loss of the image I portrayed of her to protect her in life while dishonoring my own truth about our relationship.

It was very freeing to let go of a false image and finally embrace the truth of my pain from our relationship.

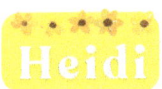

How do you honor those who have transitioned? In the last few years, whenever I see or hear or feel something related to those who have transitioned, I smile and say hi to them out loud. I'll hear a Billy Joel song in Walgreens and say "Hi dad."

Or when I'm playing cards with my son, I'll smile and tell him about my great aunt and the epic card games we played with peanuts and small glasses of ginger ale.

It's these small moments that make me feel connected to these ancestors and help pass down stories to my son.

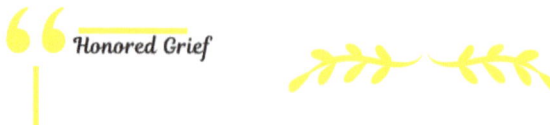

Alex Aguilar

What I have come to learn in loneliness was grief and sorrow but also growth and healing. The sorrow I experienced filled every fiber of my bone with this pain and solitude. It occupied every corner of my mind. Loosing friends and being in solitude numbed the reality of who I was. I was cheerful, and life was great, but when being abandoned by my friends, my life turned from day to night. Though this experience was strong, it did not break me, but instead, it shaped me.

I learned from this experience and I understand holding on to the pain and resentment did not allow me to grow or move forward. In my faith I found healing and I learned to let go of all the pain and suffering I dragged each day of my life.

I know suffering is inevitable but whether I'm with friends or not I understood that the important thing is to not put my happiness in others but to be happy being with myself and when possible, sharing that happiness with others.

Company is great and so is solitude. That balance is important to find and it just takes one step at a time.

"

Julie Neale
Founder, Coach and Community Builder at Mother's Quest
www.mothersquest.com

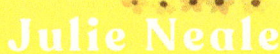

Through laughter and tears, I recorded a special solo cast to officially close out Season Six of the Mother's Quest Podcast so I can begin again. It felt like part of my healing to share my stories with you and I'm hopeful that there may be something in these reflections that can be meaningful and healing for you too.

Death is one of the few things we can all count on in our lives. And yet it's one of the things we are most reluctant to talk about.

I hope this exploration of my experience during my father's death, and the lessons I learned, might support you to open yourself to conversations about death. In so doing, you'll open yourself more fully to life and love.

"There is nothing so whole as a broken heart" – a quote I cut out in a magazine while working on my vision board the other day. It resonated immediately.

There were so many people, whose wisdom, compassion, and caring made moving through this painful process not only bearable but at times beautiful. Thank you. Thank you. Thank you. You helped me and my family stay whole and I am so grateful."

Lessons To Guide You Through the Death of a Loved One

In this episode, I walk you through the eight lessons I learned through my father's death, my grief, and most importantly– my love for my Dad and my family.

1) Look for the Signs
2) Find Your Guides
3) Closure Can be Healing
4) Lean Into Your Rituals. Make Them Your Own.
5) Let Laughter In and Invite the Possibility that the Unexpected Can be a Gift
6) Release Perfectionism and Shame
7) Open Your Heart and Ride the Waves
8) Have the Conversations

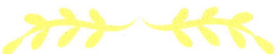

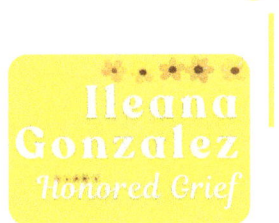

Ileana
Gonzalez
Honored Grief

I would like to share a memory of Mr Ayala.
I remember him always so excited to the days Angel would be going home to the Velasquez family and how caring and loving he was with Angel. A true meaning of "blood doesn't make you family." Angel loved him very much and from as long as I can remember he has always called him grandpa.

And not just anyone allows someone else's child to call them "grandpa." This man was a very joyful and upbeat man from when I was able to see and hear as well as the moments, I was able to witness with my family when both families would unite. I will forever be grateful in my heart that my son was able to share fun and beautiful moments with Mr.Ayala.

What grief has taught me is that grief doesn't only happen in death. You grieve even the ones alive. Why? Because there are relationships in life you may never know why they just disappeared or have shifted away.

There is relationships you miss and wish where still a there but yet are not. You miss being able to talk to someone who is dear to your heart but have chosen or just slowly stayed away. You miss the laughter's and jokes. You miss so much.

Grief has taught it's better to grieve the ones who are

gone because in the end they're in a better place. But its ten times harder to grieve the ones alive and are so close yet so far.

Grieving a process of finding self-strength and love. As well as learning to be grateful and blessed for what you already have in front of you.

For the things you once wished for even if they're not exactly as you planned.

——𝟗𝟗

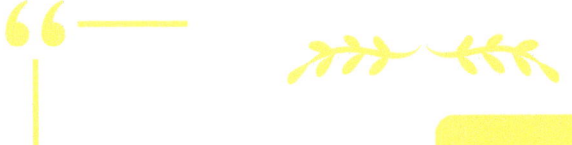

Angel Velasquez

Grief to me is about lessons learned, like mostly with friends. Time is never promised, you have to appreciate what you have while you have it. There is no time promised between you and anybody. You have to embrace it while you can. And with death, don't be sad they are gone- be happy the time you got to have with them.

Some people don't get the time you did. I don't mean I don't get sad, but I am trying to be glad about the time I had with them. Yes, I wish certain things but at the end of the day I don't want their memory to live off of what I wish—I want the memory to live off of what we did have.

Those memories, of my grandma and grandpa are what holds the place in my heart.

Athena, Age 6

Grief is making memory boxes and telling what you are scared of.
I miss hugging my grandma martha whenever we would visit each other. I want to tell her that I love her.

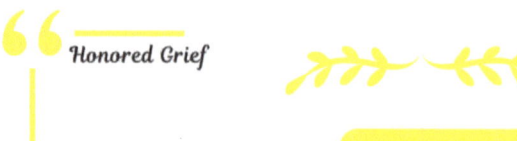

Iris Ayala-Velasquez

One lesson I learned from grief was that the grieving process isn't linear and is different for everyone. I also learned that all emotions are on the table , one minute you can feel sad and the next you are angry -ect. In my opinion it's a feeling of shock and unable to express emotions and being treated unfairly.

What supports me is having people I can talk about it withand honor/remember them in my own way. You can heal traumatic experiences and deaths but always will grieve or mourn in some kind of way.
I wish I spent more time with my grandma martha.

Leo, Age 12

I don't know what grief has taught me. Grief has made me feel grief. It almost put me in depression. I know that because I know what I feel and what I felt. This has to do with the passing of my grandma. I don't remember when my grandpa passed, I was too young. I do not feel like the grief support groups that hospice provided helped me in the grief I was feeling, because it was a group setting.

One thing my grandma taught me I will always remember is how to say thank you, your welcome and count to 10 in Spanish. It is important to me because she taught me that before anyone else did.

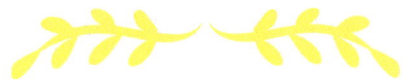

For all who shared, thank you. I know each of you personally and have so much to say in return.

But these shares are not for me to speak back to (unless you'd like to conversate, then of course, I am open.) These shares are for me to listen and share and feel. These shares are for the readers to connect with.

These shares are for you as the writers. I am so honored you said yes to the invitation to be included in this way. Thank you for your vulnerability, honesty, courage, and voice.

Before I answer each question myself. Let me be transparent in saying and naming, sometimes my answers change. Depending on the moment and time, it may not always be the same. So, in this moment is how I am answering and reflecting.

How do you honor those who have transitioned?

-Going to the cemetery and cleaning up the space, decorating, having a picnic, gathering, chalk art, being.

-Celebrating anniversaries and birthdays. Including them in holidays and important milestones by having them in pictures or on shirts- things like that

-Writing about them. Speaking about them. Tears, laughter, sharing memories.

altars
-I have made sweaters with pictures and quotes, pillows that are full body images or other kinds, ornaments, picture books with pictures and quotes, cards with pictures and quotes, blankets with pictures, canvases of pictures, cups with pictures, digital frames that play videos and pictures,
-enjoying recipes loved ones enjoyed.

What lessons has grief taught you?

Grief has taught me to be intentional with those living. That I can honor those living, in the same or similar ways I do those who have passed. Creating certain things does not have to just be because of a passing.

-That it is ok to be ok
-It is ok, to not be ok. To take my time with grief and how I feel.
-That every loss might have similar things, maybe you can prepare "better" in some ways but there will always be the unexpected and new things to navigate and learn.

It has taught me that with the passing of my mother-in-law, This journey feels a lot different. It feels like I have to bite my tongue, It feels like I don't have a say, It feels like walls are up and the grief is not just mine

What does your grief want you to know?

-Right now my grief wants me to know that it is ok it looks and feels different with the passing of my mother-

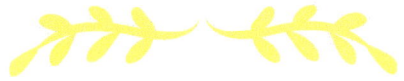

in-law than that of dad.

It's ok that my dad's passing couldn't prepare me to know all I wish I could've foreseen when my mother-in-law transitioned.

---that my anger is valid

And, it wants e to embrace what's real. So that I can honor her and myself and so that I can heal.

When it comes to grief, what are you grateful for?

-I am grateful for the memories, the pictures, the videos, the Facebook words shared, words shared through cards, signatures left behind.

-I am grateful for tears of release

-I am grateful for feeling my feelings

-I am grateful for books created, healing spaces held, opportunities given from sharing my truth and being with my journey

-I am grateful for traditions I have created

What is grief?

Grief is that sadness of a memory that brings you to a stop, a pause, a reflection. That memory that brings a smile and also a knowing that -you can't make more memories with the person who has left earthside.

Grief is that heartache and heartbreak that can feel crippling and also so empowering to keep going. Grief is a journey.

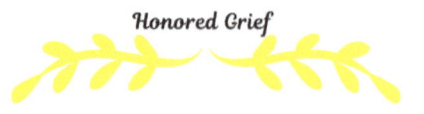

What does it mean to grieve?

For me it means to allow myself to feel whats real but not to live there. At least not forever. It also means to me that it is not "black or white" and it is not "linear"- it is a journey. It is forever, in a sense that it is a part of me. It will come and go and show itself in different ways.

How does it feel in your body and show in your actions?

In this season, grief has shown up very painfully. It has shown up in constipation and enormous back pain. It has shown up in anger and nausea. It has shown up and I didn't even realize what it was until I allowed myself to give it voice and choice and recognition. It has shown up as inflammation. How do I know these things? Because I am getting to know my body and I am paying attention to my journey.

What does it feel/look like to heal while on the grief journey?

It feels and looks differently, at different times. It is moment by moment sometimes. It is a whole spectrum of realities, sometimes with many existing at once. Healing on this journey looks like not forgetting or curing, but being with.

That we are whole as we are- with the sadness, anger, grief, happiness-whatever is true.

My message to readers and writers, as we have now combined for some of this journey: You are not a product or content.

This collaboration was an intentional invitation to share stories and honor grief/healing/each other/ ourselves/ our loved ones. This collaboration was a calling from the heart, an answered call that led to something I could have never even dreamed of. Thank you all.

I then found myself being curious about what that felt like for people to reflect in that way, I wondered why they said yes to the invitation.

I wonder what it will feel like for them to read their messages and that of others once this book is in hands. So, naturally-It took a moment but I built the courage to ask some whom shared:

"If you feel called to share, I'd love to hear. Because I know this is a part of the journey and my path.

- *What did it feel like to write your message to share?*
- *How did it feel to reflect?*
- *What "made" you say yes to this invitation?"*

And some people shared:-

- It was an interesting experience. While I knew that I was in my body and I was present with myself, there was another part of me that was aware that what was coming through me was not entirely from me. It felt cathartic and clarifying. Divine appointment is why I said yes---Bernadette

- I've had a creative block especially around my words for a very long time. Sometimes that block manifests physically with health issues. It felt freeing to be able to write what grief has taught me. My grief needs to be acknowledged by me and witnessed in community. It felt validating, a huge release much needed, I said yes to sharing because it was a no brainer! I wanted to help a friend and since I'm working with grief more I felt I had to honor my journey. Iv'e grown and healed so much. I realized grief was the fertilizer to help me birth the new work I am doing now. It's overwhelming going through it but still grateful for it. -Katrina.

- It helped me get unstuck and now I have all these ideas of what I want to put out. You opened the door and now I can't stop it. I don't want to stop. I feel free to allow myself to be, to be seen. To be me. Anonymous.

- It felt like a part of my brain unlocked because I don't usually write like that. And I like what I wrote. I feel good about it and proud. Anonymous.

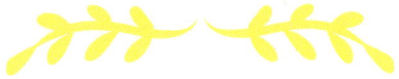

- I don't have a dream to write an entire book but it felt nice to share my story short and concise in this way and I loved it. ---Jasmin

- For more than a decade I couldn't write, not the way I was able to for this. Now I am inspired in the work I do and how I want to show up. Anonymous.

- I said yes because I don't talk often about my thoughts on grief. It's hard to think about, let alone write about. I realize I don't reflect on this enough because I was in tears just writing what I did. -Syhara.

I never talk about my feelings, to anyone. I never even spend that much time with myself. I shared because I love Lena and I love what her writings have done for me and my heart and my life. I am sharing because I now see and feel what sharing my experiences maybe can do for someone else, even just for myself.

Now I kind of get what you mean when you say "if you can write a fb post, you can write a book" I am inspired to do so much more and I see that with the right question, the right connection- sometimes things can happen effortlessly.
Thank you.

I share my original Facebook posts and journal pages and writings- as they are when they were written. Yes, with typos, errors, and all.

I share this way both on purpose and with purpose. I choose not to have an editor come in and change anything. I want to share in this real way. I feel like this way of being is who I am and have always been, it is a part of my purpose here on earth-to show up in this way.

And so, I also share people's writings (who have given permission here)—also in their true authentic ways.
I believe in being transparent, open, and real. I do it for my peace and heart but also maybe it will inspire others to do the same

.

This book is yours, however you choose to engage with it.

No judgement, just gratitude to connect in any way.

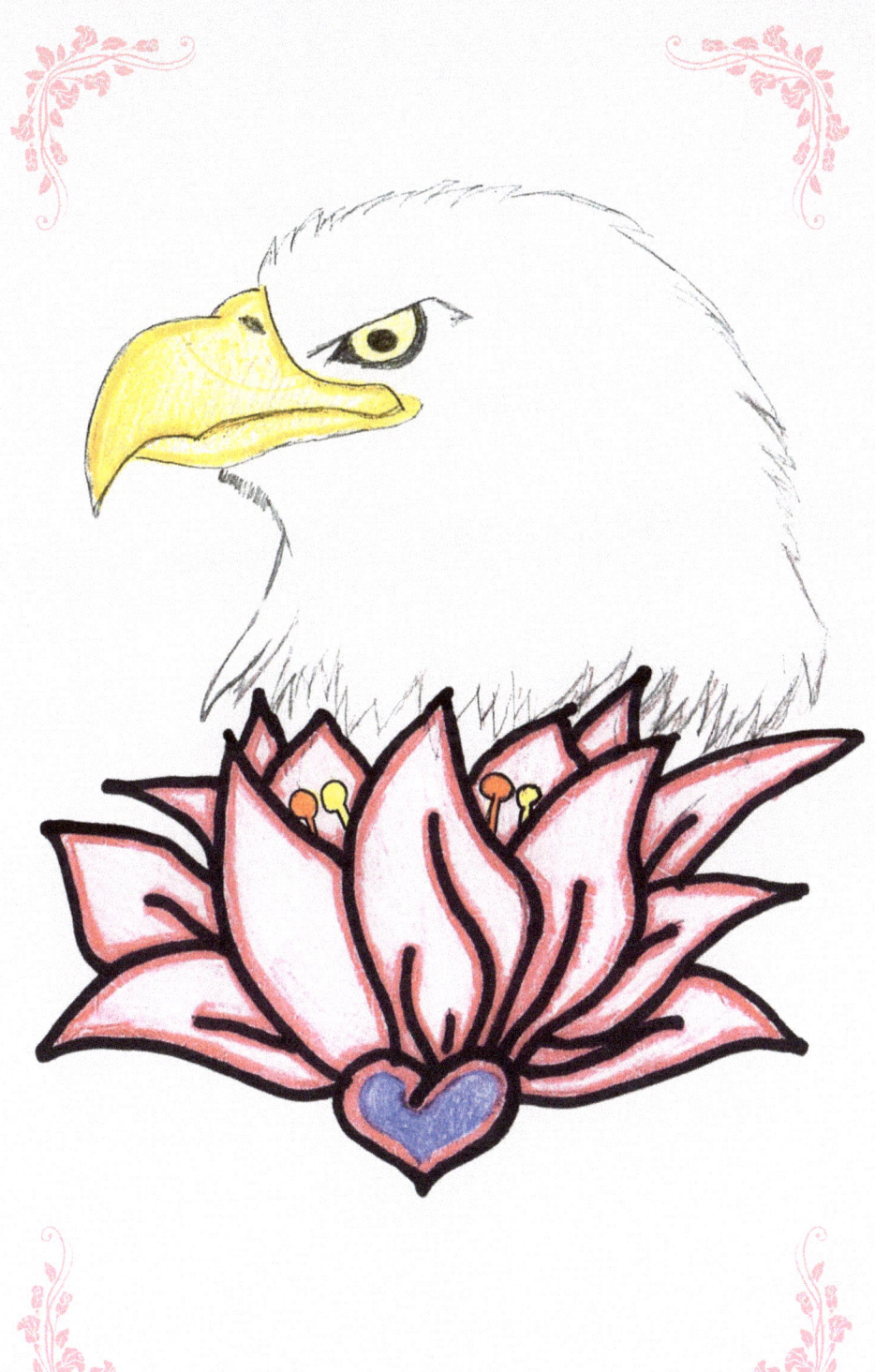

Chapter

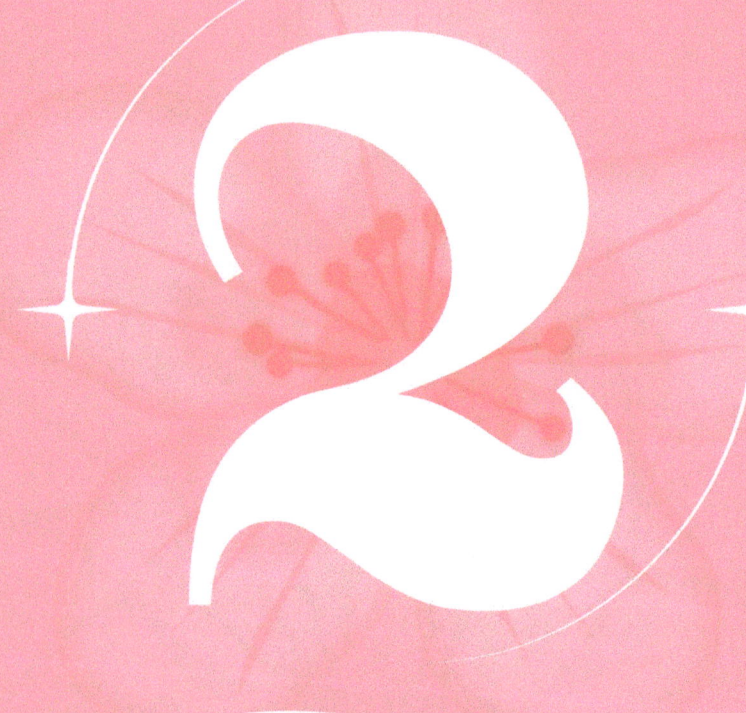

2

Healing While Hurting

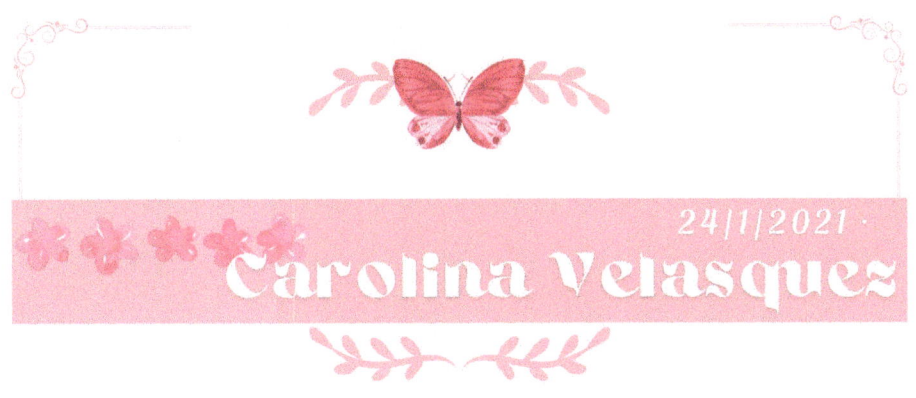

Carolina Velasquez

Writing/Publishing a book has been on my mind and heart since the 4th grade.
Over the last few years, I found myself talking about it out loud more.

Last year I accepted an invitation to The Tiny Book Course. I asked if there was a scholarship option but there was not. This meant I had to borrow money, use saved/bill money for other things I would have to be ok to go without....

I was able to pay for early bird pricing and afford the cheapest option of having to do much on my own. (classic level). Iwas skeptical about what I paid. How can anyone guarantee this book will get done? How can this "cheapest" price be the only cost? Surely more costs will arise, what will I do then?

The fact that someone I trust recommended this course to me, the fact that she too was thinking of taking this journey, the fact that she then had an affiliate connection---made it all worth it.

I knew I wanted to make this dream real and wait no longer, 2020 would be it for me.
It was exactly the kind of support, opportunity, and

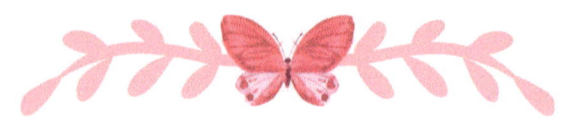

way I would want to create my first book: with live sessions, weekly email support, contest, and prizes, in community with some mothersquest members, with a timeframe, all the recourses to keep forever, hearing from people who took the course before....

My mindset of 2020 was "I already know what not trying looks like, I want to know what trying will look like. what will taking risks bring me. what doors will open."

I knew all the things I wanted in my book.
It would be about my dad, about my journey since losing him. It would be a poetry book, with reflections.
I wanted to have quotes from him, the kids, I wanted pictures, I wanted pages open for journaling and reflections, I wanted to share what helped me/what i learned and what I still wish.

I had people I wanted to thank, I knew I wanted my husband and kids involved, I knew i wanted to honor people, i wanted a biography of my dad and me, I wanted to talk about the years before cancer-when he died, the time after, i wanted to share memories, I wanted my mother-in-law to pick a prayer, i wanted the serenity prayer, i wanted to add the poem my dad had in his wallet(not everything made it in.)

was it going to be just for me, for family, for the world? what would that really mean? Facebook has always been my diary, my blog, my photo album.

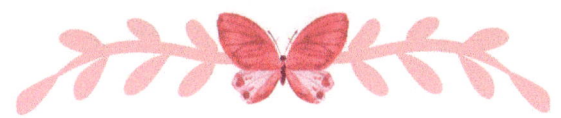

Earlier in the year of 2020 I knew I was going to do something with my life that would involve the lotus flower.

I have always had a connection to "smile now, cry later" cry now, smile later. The title could have even been Hurting while healing.

Creating this book was important to me. Because something inside of me was calling me to do this. I needed to do this for me, to answer my inner voice, to follow my heart and to continue healing me.

I wanted to do this because I wanted to show my family, my children that dreams do come true and I wanted them to be proud of me. I wanted to feel proud of me. I want to help the world, in whatever way I can. People have told me in the past how my words have helped them and that matters to me.

I had nothing to lose, only something to gain. Of course, the fear of "losing" out on invested money and time. The fear of not getting it done, it not being good enough

I knew I wanted an ISBN , I wanted to be and feel like a real author, I wanted a paperback book.
Holding my book is the feeling I want, a dream I could see but didn't know how.
Do I want it to create income? that would be nice but what I truly wanted was it to create healing.
I know my journey is mine, no copyright. So no worries

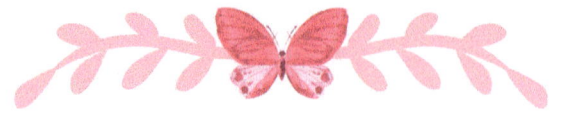

there. I had most of the content already.

I knew I wouldn't have chapters but I had a "way" of structure in mind. I debated on "who am I to decide such things? has it been done before? Can I just follow my heart even if it's never been done?

I wanted to write, I wanted to enjoy the process, I wanted to stay true to my vision and heart and I wanted to get it done! Make it real.
I made the choice to embark on this journey, I wanted it to feel good-not like a burden.

I have spent the last few years really working on me from the inside out. This was another part in investing in me and my healing, in not just learning to dream again-but in making my dream real.

I want my reader to know my dad, to get to know me, to have a chance to reflect. I want my reader to leave with knowing that its ok to not be ok...and its ok to be ok. That wherever you are in life is where you are meant to be and "perfection" isn't necessary. We are all 'perfect" as is, errors and all. Typos and all. Our stories matter. Sharing matters.

Healing happens through the painful stuff and it is an on-going process. I hope you can find healing in your own journey. I want my reader to be able to relate and feel connected---even if I am so personal about my own story.

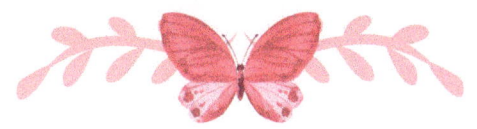

18|11|2023·

An older woman saw the title "healing while writing" and flipped through kinda quickly
"My husband passed away in august"

I'm so sorry.... I barley had the urge to say...

(Hands over her mouth, her hands shaking) She couldn't bear to look anymore, tears coming as she walked to a friend to lean on, gather herself and continue at the event of pop up tables...

I just wanted to hug her and offer gifts....

Grief is like this moment. It hits when you don't expect.
And it's never the "right time or place"
and there's not enough permission or space.

But what if there was?

It is so clear to me, if I do not sell a single book today, I was here for this.
A reminder of my calling to hold spaces for grief.
That something as simple as a title, could be so impactful and powerful.
That hearing someone and letting them know you heard them- can be more than enough.

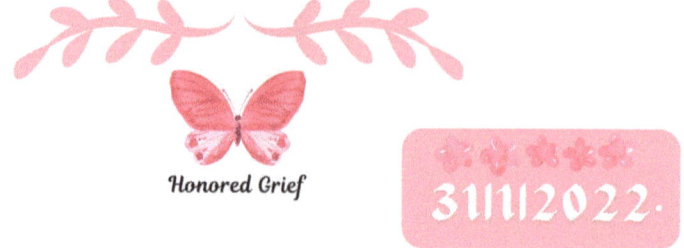

I am feeling so in alignment. With my purpose, my direction, my story, my pieces of me, my path.

Today I had several moments of just pure bliss.
Today I met for about 40minutes with a soul care sister. I feel like we both helped each other. It was just a normal check in and time as friends. Somewhere in there I felt my coach side just tap in, like fully tap in and it feels so good to listen, to reflect, to celebrate and support another person.

I don't have a niche. I am just me.
and I am still able to help others.
It felt empowering, exciting, and just a sense of pure happiness.

I had a moment with my uncle kirk. He is halfway through my second book. I shared he is reading the unrevised edition and he said, it's ok. That he is enjoying it.
"It can apply to anyone. ages 12-50 (just as example)"
"You get the points across. your style of writing is you."

"I'm gonna order two copies, one for me and a friend. "
His friend heard him speak about it, and wants to read!"It has potential"
"It made me rethink of something I have been writing and written"

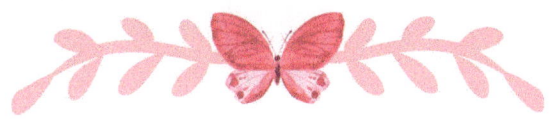

"This could have had many titles and been relevant to many things, it is relatable"

our hug, his support, his love. I felt like I was hugging not just a dad. but a father figure for me. He always has been. In so many ways these lessons in this book are ones he has always taught me and brought to my life.

I am so forever grateful to him and for him.

Day 3 of coming home to your true nature, manifesthouse.
The lotus.
It is 4 pm but the way the day is unfolding resonates.
Last night I saw the interior design of my next book and of course right away I am drawn in by the lotus illustration on the cover and what it means to be in grief but to find healing through writing.
Journaling, reflecting, expressing,

I went to get x-rays this morning, only to be told they couldn't find my referral. So, they didn't get done. I felt like we wasted time, gas, energy and now I was carrying the feelings of failure, continued pain without solution, frustration and more.

I talked it out, well I talked through it during counseling. Hopefully will get some answers or direction soon.
I feel like February has been this for me. I have been pulling myself out of the hard stuff and every time I pull out- I feel like I get thrown back down. But each fall or challenge just adds on to what was before, instead of "get better"

The car is still not fixed, my book still incomplete, habits and routines still not created, goals undone, the good is there but the bad is what feels most center stage.

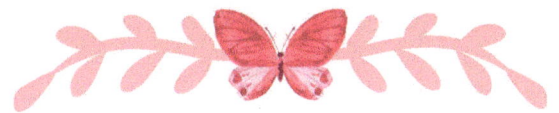

Today, even in pain. I decided to finally use our upholstery cleaner. 11am-1:40pm I was cleaning our couch. Two rounds of clean to dirty water. Because I do not want my husband to do more work after work, I want something crossed off the to do list.

I am tired of seeing things the way they are when I want change and I can change them. So, I went for it. Asked for help from my oldest at times.
Learning the machine, listening to my body and pushing it. When cushions would dry, I would see stains still and go back for a second, even third cleaning.

And still, some of them need more time. but I said enough was enough. I let the help be enough, the work be enough and the time be enough.
for now. The sun was out, it was windy. thankful for that support.

I am taking the lesson that some scars, stains, marks---take time to clean or heal. Even after several sessions, lots of time and support. Sometimes things don't just heal or get fixed. Sometimes it takes more and more.
And that's ok.

Not everyone will notice the hard work that was put into the parts that are now cleaner.
Not everyone will see the clean (healing) parts because of the stains still left.

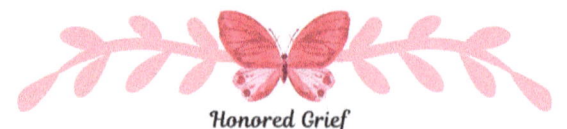

Honored Grief

Some might feel they can do better job.
Some will say just throw it all away, buy fresh, start again.

The amount of dirt that came through, you never would have been able to tell how deep the stains go.
You may never know the stains that remain are cleaner than they once were.
Some will only see stains.
Some will see character or stories to be shared.

But I know.
You know.
We know the work we put in.
We know the struggles we face.
We know what it took to get to where we are.
We know the difference.

Will you be extra cautious now that you put in this work?
Does it not matter because you have a machine to help for the next situation?

Maybe this time I won't wait years before cleaning.
Maybe next time I'll get to the spills and what not before they take such big holds.
Maybe next time we will use this nifty machine for the car.

11/11/2023·

Writing a book is "hard."
It's simple and yet layered. Because we are human and we deal with so many thoughts and emotions and paradigms and everything.

Add the layer of writing about grief or trauma. and it's all extra to the process.

You can end up at a standstill. a roadblock. a pause. and not understand why. the trauma and pain, re-living anything. sometimes we store those memories and feelings and energies---even with healing. sometimes we feel it again and process again and just don't want to go through it again.

So, we shut down. I like to think it's just our bodies telling us to take a break, breathe and then get back to it. but take care of you during that in-between time

It'll come back, or come in how it's meant to. because it's your journey. you probably just needed a little break.

When I find myself frustrated in any of this writing process. I go back to my why. why am I doing this. remind myself of what's important. take a minute to do something that brings me joy and don't force the process.

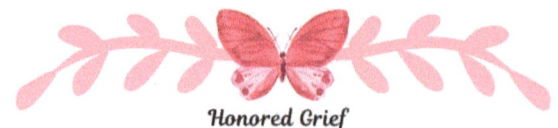

Remember to celebrate how far you have come. all the writing you have done. Where you are at. celebrate yourself for all it took you to be here because it took you being born, having those experiences, and now telling the story. never forget to celebrate your progress. because all the steps matter. and the work you are doing is heavy and powerful.

I had several people give opinions and it brought me fear. I went back to my "why." and back to my heart. Following my heart brought peace and miracles. no-matter what anyone else thought.
I like to take what people say and think of how it can help me know more of what I want, maybe even lead me to changes to help certain things not become issues.

It's all for reasons that make sense in the end. sometimes I am better at getting to things and telling the story when I go backwards.
Several times I started working backwards and it helped me get the vision I wanted.

Follow your hearts lead.

5/11/2023.

As I continue working on creating book number 6. I am reminded of lessons learned that continue to return

*A free title upload would have been great to take advantage of last month.
It would have saved me $50

*My ultimate goal and deadline is January 21st.
In honor of my dad's anniversary

*When writing, reflecting, and dealing with grief. In any way or form and it's layers. It takes more than just "the work."
It takes energy, brings up emotions, sometimes you pause and don't realize why.
This isn't just about creating a book or journal.
It is so much more than that.
It is about honoring loved ones, honoring myself, my process, my pace, my truths.

It is about taking my time. Not about rushing a good deal. Because I have learned in the past- that sometimes rushing for a good deal, can lead to paying more financial costs to fix things in the end and take longer for the final product and vision to be.

I do not have a full vision on what I want this book/journal to be.

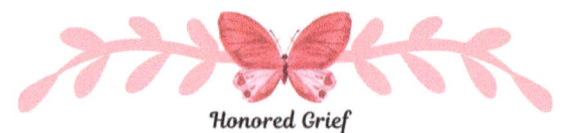

I do have my goal that this week I want to be done writing so I can pass it off to someone to get it print ready.
I will make it to all of my goals.
but I am happy during workout and meditation this morning that I was reminded of taking my time.

That success is what we define it to be.
That I know I can do this.
I will do this.
and I just want to love it.

I do not need to compare it to my first book, which I love so much.
It will be beautiful, perfect, and powerful in its own way.
It will be what it needs to be.
what it's meant to be.

............in all honesty. I spent only a couple of days really writing and putting it together so much.
most days for the last few months have been not working on it, not typing, not doing.
they have been spent meditating, crying, working on me and all of my feelings and thoughts and life. and that is ok.

Sometimes the work is done when we aren't "working" on the goal.
sometimes the work is done in-between the deadlines and what not.

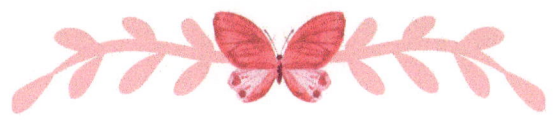

Kind of like that dash between the dates of life and death.....
So much happens in between. and so much happens beyond.

Allow yourself time. allow yourself time to be real. time to feel, to flow and be.

261312023·

"I've been reading your book, I read it on the train or outside. I cried a few times. I won't write, my thoughts are mine-I know what they are. I don't need it to fall in the wrong hands. But I love the pictures" - Uncle Lu

"it's kind of like the first book"
yeah, similar but with writing pages. So, people can take time to reflect, get creative, write whatever they want. Sometimes we gain clarity or healing from writing.

I appreciate any time someone shares anything with me.
whether this journal gets written in, read or both or just looked at. Whatever the case, it serves its purpose.

"You made your money, what does it matter if I write in it or not?"
it doesn't.
It is just an option.
The book is for however it serves, whomever it is meant to serve.

It is not about the money.
what's its purpose then?
well....

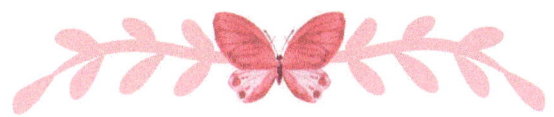

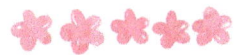

- This book is about speaking the names and sharing the faces of people I love. My bloodline. People who matter to my heart. My ancestors.
- It is about life beyond death
- It is about living in my purpose
- My purpose to be open and honest. My purpose to be real and raw. My purpose to be transparent. My purpose of sharing me, so that others can build courage to share their stories. So that others can know and feel it's ok to not be perfect.
- To continue the narrative and knowing, that grief and healing are ongoing. There is no timeline or timeframe or one way through.
- Because writing, reflecting, taking time to be with my thoughts and emotions in this way, is part of who I am.
- Because I don't aim to inspire but I leave space for it to maybe be. By sharing me.
- This is my heart-work.
- This is a way of income. A way of my family living dreams.
- This is one way I honor those I love, both living and no longer.
- This is one way I heal.

Honored Grief

In life mastery tonight we were asked a few questions. what agreement is speaking to you this month/in this moment

"Have fun and faith" is what has been and is speaking to me.
So much, that today when I asked myself how I could be in more alignment with me-the answer was make time for the park with the kids.

But tonight, as we got home, my youngest went for a late nap and started breathing weird and coughing.
"It was cold out, it's because we let her go to the park" feeling a little guilt, I then decided nope. It wasn't the park. we were there like 10minutes. she needs time out, play, fun, walking, exercise. And I stepped into my alignment and faith, I am standing by it.

What area are you focusing on this month?

I said health and wellness. along with fun and faith.
I say this because working out has been on my to do list forever. Maybe if I made it fun, with music. I want more plant based because that's just what my mind body and soul are into right now and want to explore.

I want more water, because I know that makes me feel best. I want to live in and speak my truth more. I want more shakes because when I was doing that,

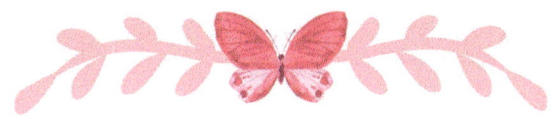

I loved how it made me feel. I want more engagement with kids.

Our youngest isn't feeling good in this moment, she is laying on me and I am in this meeting. I am multi-tasking but soaking in this moment. I couldn't hold our oldest daughter in this way when she wasn't feeling good earlier this week.

More fun has been on my mind and heart: park, biking, baking, music, games. faith has been on my mind: church, step into, speak about it, say what I need to say. Trust

What are you celebrating? What is a wi
Today I had so much time, that wasn't planned for. Many cancelled meetings and things. So, I told myself I would do all the things I haven't yet. like working out and work on my book. (Perhaps if I invite in more fun, then the book process and working out will be more do-able

But then I was upset at myself that I didn't.
I re-evaluated what I did make time for and now I decided I am going to celebrate it and the wins. I am celebrating the time. The time alone, the time to shower- alone and listen to music and be with my thoughts.

***Sickness does not have to mean we did something wrong or be about guilt or shame.

Sickness can be here to show us, all we are doing right. It can be here to test our faith and growth and learning. To lean into what we believe to be true and know to be true. to step into growth and faith.

Sickness doesn't mean "bad mom" or bad parent.
Yes, it could be an eye-opener of what we can do better, connect dots to what may have led here
Or, maybe people just get sick sometimes.

Maybe it means we need to pause. We need to focus on rest. We need to put the phones down and spend that time to cuddle and be love and support and feel the same in return.
These challenging moments in time remind me of my humanness and that I still fear some things and it shows me how far I have come and how much more I trust me.

Tap into what spirit, the universe, GOD and life is trying to tell you.
trying to show you. trying to teach you.
Sometimes we get the same messages, in different ways- until we do something different for different results.
Sometimes, it is time to change.
Sometimes, it is time to listen.
Whatever message is for you, is-for you

My head has clarity, my heart feels peace. and now I am complete with my reflection, writing and sharing.

18|5|2021·

With each book created, I learn so much.
About the people I hire to support in certain parts of creating.
I learn about me, what I am capable of. What I want to learn and what I already know.
I learn about what is my "good enough" and what is not.

I learn what I would do different next time.
This 4th time is no different.
I remind myself that no version has to stay the way it is forever, if I don't want it to.
I can update, change, and revise any time. I can add or take-away anything at any time I choose.
I do have choices.

Something about me and this journey is I take pride in my truth. I love my authenticity. I do not always like or love my errors and mistakes but I love sending the message that you can create something, such as a book and becoming an author- without needing to be "perfect."

You can make your dreams real. You can continue to dream. You can begin again. You can do different, be different and you will grow.
It takes courage to put yourself out there, especially with all of your imperfections.

But I also believe we can send messages to others that inspire them. and We create messages for ourselves.

*"Delivered" got that text and I went running, huge smile.
I wanted to love it.
I knew it was not my complete vision.
When I hired someone from fiverr to do the interior format + create to cover/back … that process was also not my complete vision.
This person decided to "help edit" when I didn't ask. I am now seeing things that were changed that I do not like.

I see many typos, a few repeats.
I love that her background art makes the pages nicer.
(Iris said it gives coloring book vibes and I love that feeling of being able to color and write on the pages honestly.)
The spacing for writing could be smaller.
The fonts are different sizes and the spacing she chose; I do not love.
I do not love the table of contents.
There are no page numbers.
Our names not on the spine.

There are some prompts said twice. But I approved this because I thought it could be nice for people to be able to answer some questions twice, or have more space to write.
Maybe I should have made the pages white instead of

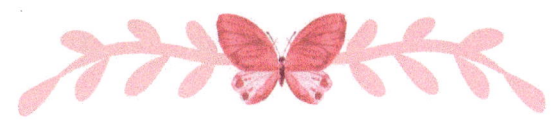

crème. As usual, I am going through this real-life copy and making my edits with my pen.

I told myself, with my last book that I would do the interior myself.
But I saw a free title upload and "rushed again"
And paid someone from fiverr
And rushed through to get the free upload- even not loving it but not realizing all the errors.
In the end- it is on me because I had to approve the e-proof and I did without making further changes.
I was in such a rush that so much was last minute and missed and seen as "good enough" to get it done.

I appreciate the person for wanting to help and having good intentions.
I thank my daughter for her help.
I thank ingramspark for the free title upload.
I thank me for getting a book done so quickly- even if imperfect.

I purposely did not have an editor because I did not want anyone changing my vision and my style and words and messages- but somehow that still happened. However, an editor for repetition and small words like "its" would have been great to have and catch.
We will always be hard on ourselves, I know I am.
Others will always have judgement.
What matters to me, is that I got it done.

What matters to me- is that I am happy.
What matters to me is that I am growing and learning and continuing to create.

I guess I am rolling with this unpolished authentic me. I share all of this because I want people to know the very real parts of this process and journey. I like to share my truth and the "behind the scenes." I know I am not perfect and I hope my imperfections inspire you to be easier on yourself and to "just do it"- whatever your heart is calling you to do.

16|12|2023·

Opportunity did not just come for no reason,
Why not go for it...so let's write this email and press send....

Hello, my name is Carolina Ayala- but I mostly go by Lena. I am a mother of 4, a wife and more.
My mother-in-law passed from cancer a little over a year ago now. My dad passed away due to cancer in 2014. I have experienced grief and loss even before these dates of passing.

When it comes to grief, I am still in it. I do not think it has an end date. I feel it is a journey that is both painful and something I am grateful for. I wrote and self-published my first book "Healing while hurting" in 2020 and "Healing while writing" in 2023.

I share this to share, through and with my grief- I became an author.

For me, my creative experiences come from this journey. I have been a writer of poetry since the 4th grade, I have always turned to reflection and writing as my ways to cope and heal and express. I also turn to pictures I have taken. Spoken word is something I turn to when I am processing.

Before my book was made, I had spent all the years since my fathers passing - documenting my journey.

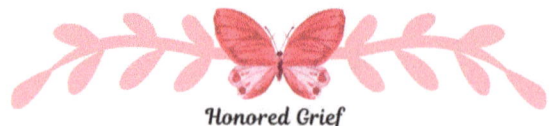

Honored Grief

I did this on fb and in journals and then turned it into my first ever book. This month I created a grief and gratitude card deck, I also plan to turn that into another book "Honored grief" - journal prompts.
I have held several grief spaces this year, virtually. This journey is on-going and continues to unfold.

I may be rambling now, but grief has brought me many lessons and experiences I never once thought for myself. Thank you for your time

Honored Grief

You may feel behind, unaccomplished, lost, stuck, scared....
You may feel so many things. And it is ok.
I encourage you to share your truth and journey.
Someone out there often feels the same, someone out there might have needed to hear what you had to say.
By sharing, you create release, relief, and growth. You create courage, hope and trust.

I have been feeling a whirlwind of emotions while writing this book.
Someone today asked me about it. Asked me how I was doing it. Said she had always wanted to write a book and asked if I could share the link of the course I am going through.
She told me "So many people often think, I want to write a book, and they don't do it-you are doing it! you did it!"

Whether someone hits like, love or leaves a comment-people are watching and reading what you share.
You never know who you are inspiring.
You never know the connections you are making when you are open. As I was writing this post I then came across this next part, and it all ties in so well......

*Julie posted this:

What are some of YOUR favorite things? What work in

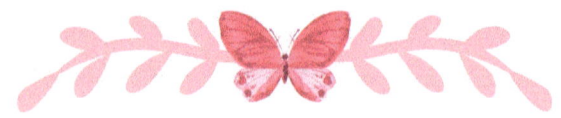

your world is lighting you up? What collaborations are giving you fuel to keep doing what you do? Would love to hear. And I love questions like this and time to reflect and dig a little deeper.

Some of my favorite things are being with my family. Embracing being home with the kids, although I am not "working" I am enjoying being home and helping with school. I love writing, taking photos and creating special gifts for people. So much work in the world is lighting me up: I am so thankful for the teachers(I am thankful to have been one, to be one- even if I am technically not being paid for it right now), I am thankful for the investment in chiropractic help-all I am learning and feeling and how it is helping change me for the better,

I am so thankful for all of the coaches in my life and for me being able to help others, although I do not yet call myself a "coach". The fuel to keep going and doing what I do is gratitude. Every day I have so much gratitude for all that's in my life. Right now, I am so thankful to be a part of mothers quest and the tiny book course, I am so thankful to be in soul care with barb klein and the courageous life society with jessica stong. I have so many people in my life right now who make me happy/healthy and strong and I am so thankful. ....I really love getting up, making my bed and starting my day that way-setting intention.

Something has really stuck with me from soul care

Honored Grief

Monday.

We often think of our future self as someone years from now. But our future self can be us 5 minutes from now. How do you help create your future self? What are you doing now to support your future self?

Even so much as waking up and making your bed, how that helps you feel through the day and sets you up for success at night.

I made a post before this one about how I specifically set up my weekly chiropractic visits for Thursday because I wanted to start off my morning with self care and happiness on thankful Thursdays. because for me, that feels good.

I started thinking what else makes me feel good and as I was hungry and wanted to indulge, I made a shaekology drink-because that makes me feel good. It makes me feel healthier, it makes me feel proud and accomplished and I enjoy starting my day this way and feeling this way.

How can you bring some happiness to your morning or day today?

What fills you with high vibrations?

22/11/2019.

Julie posted

What meaning or lessons do you want to claim from your E.P.I.C. Life this week?

AND/OR

What are you noticing you're grateful for? Perhaps even grateful for in the midst of challenge?

Share a lesson learned or gratitude from your week

So of course, I wanted to reflect and share

I absolutely love this whole post. What amazing gifts to share with us, how lucky are we to have you and all you bring to our lives. I missed the earlier posts so I am only just now starting today but I have definitely learned lessons and am grateful for so much every day. Every day I end my night before bed with "thankful grateful blessed" and every day I name struggles/challenges/pains and the gratitude through it all, the lessons learned and growth and hopes to continue on. This week has been one heck of a week. Appointments were missed-whether canceled by me or the other end-whether I stuck to commitment even when I did not want to. I faced a lot of situations by challenging my anxiety in hopes it will help me in the future. I learned things will work out and they wont, really to just be ok with that and not beat myself up about coulda/ woulda /shoulda/ didn't. Looking forward was placed on hold to enjoy "right now" and those days I knew to look forward to are here in the

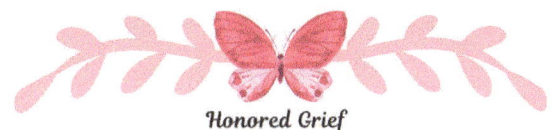

blink of an eye regardless. Every day is something to look forward to. I learned re-arranging the house and de-cluttering really makes me feel better and it makes my family feel better as well. I am grateful for the groups I am apart of such as mothers quest and surrendered healing and many others. I am grateful for the community I have been a part of that keeps on growing. I am thankful for feedback and support when asked for or not. I am thankful to have so many loving people in my life whether through social media or not. I am thankful for social media keeping connections and making new ones. I am thankful for writing prompts.

We took risks asking to call our oldest last night, it took asking with fear , fear of rejection. I can keep going. Daily I am full of gratitude-so to sum up the week, there is a lot. but thank you for the time to reflect on the week as a whole instead of me only reflecting daily. I am thankful for mothers quest birthday coming up and julies message about how it was her birthday gift to herself- it really locked in the feeling of what's next for me-over the summer I had a goal to get something done and I didn't and I now made my goal and felt it right in my heart to make a gift for myself and others to complete this project by mothers day (because that is when the idea came about) to create a grandma book based on my mom and kids.

I am thankful for you Julie. I am full of gratitude for my memories, dreams and "right now".

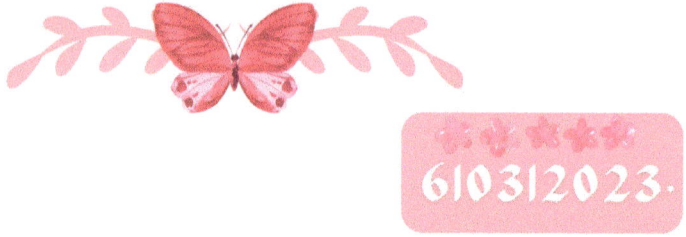

6|03|2023.

Sometimes our time to be here and present, is on a bike ride. I can put me 1st without putting others last my truth is valid and important. I am deserving of all I want. These affirmations came to me while listening to jasmine podcast episode today "unfolding."

Then, tonight at yoga. I had decided before I got there to sit off to the side. A little nervous about not wanting to be seen, I usually sit right up front and center. I noticed yesterday how much my right arm feels off and the time of the month-so I sat to the side.

Then when it was time to pull an affirmation card, my thoughts told me to be different and pull from the left instead of the right or center (for some reason I usually gravitate that way.) so I pulled from the left, I chose to go deeper (not just choose a card that was right at the top or being shown.) when I finally went in to choose, the card wouldn't just come out. Took a little work to get it out.
But right away I noticed....

It was the same card I pulled last Monday. Last Monday with no force just flow. Last Monday with intention but ease. I checked my posts from last Monday, just to see if I was right... yep, same card.

Mmmm, the message that came to me each time is how powerful our thoughts are.

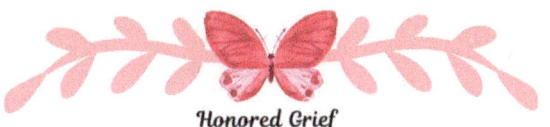

Honored Grief

To continue to creating books, writing poetry, speaking, and using my voice. But also, the power in thoughts and silence and how being present/being out in nature/being with myself- speaks to me.

The gratitude deck and podcast are callings but so is my children's book and so is homeschooling our youngest and reclaiming some of that life I created in 2020.

19|07|2021·

Waking up with the physical pain has become "everyday", again-recently. I miss the days, when I didn't miss the better days.
Hopeful.

Hello Monday, you can still be a fun-day.
You can still be magical and filled with moments that will become memories I would love to look back on, that will take me forward to where I am destined to be
My morning was more than amazing
Followed by so much living

It looks like some financial situations may soon be changing. What said pending for so long now says something else and I am so hopeful for the near future. My heart is racing, but GOD wasn't ready for the full effect yet...calling on my patience and to really re-connect with my intentions and purpose before getting the goodies.

My signed book arrived today and I already started reading "Stress-free prosperity by sneha jhanb, exactly what I need for where I am with life right now
*I pre-cooked meat yesterday for today. I re-deemed myself with my rice, this time flowing from within instead of trying to create what I think I have to for others...turned out way better now.
Soul-care was amazing as always. tonight, I feel so honored and surprised when our coach decided and

asked to use a piece from one of my facebook posts for a practice/writing prompt tonight (how to turn a stress/complain into a thank you.)
We also did an activity where we complain and vent for 2 minutes then give our gratitude for 3 minutes. I could go on forever with gratitude's, complaining was harder.

My mother-in-law, brother-in-law, sister-in-law, and nephew surprised us with a visit today. many hours together, here. unexpected and so appreciated.
my husband came for lunch with food for all, and I cooked so dinner and lunch were done for!
we enjoyed movies and time and food and i still made time for night time yoga and on camera, we decided to skip Monday night shows because of family time and yoga and rest.

As we laid down to call it a night, my brother had something happen and had to go to the ER, it was a long night. we are not sure what was wrong or is wrong but it was scary. The knots in my stomach and fear in my thoughts-were ones I haven't felt in a very long time. I was literally sick to my stomach.

It was a rough night of little sleep and not great sleep, nightmares and more. I put on the diffuser and as we were lying in bed, our youngest said my dad was here with us..........(he passed in 2014) magical, motivating, manifested, miracles and so much more.

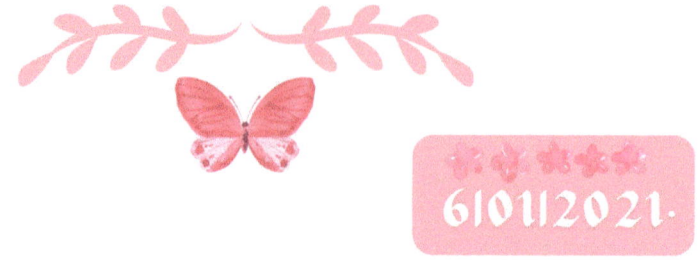

6|01|2021

I have to do a "brain dump" as Jessica Stong says "A Thought Download".

I have always known I wanted to write and publish a book. Last year Aug-Dec It all became real. The writing, thoughts, ideas, passion, desire have been in me since the 4th grade! But those last 4 months I took it past dreams and thoughts and wishes and research----I took action and I kept moving forward until it was all real, all done. Another, dream come true.

It was hard. To even figure out how to dream again. To give myself permission to dream big. To go after this without knowing how it would happen and just trust it would come together.
I have several books I want to write.
And I also want to just enjoy what this one is, will be, what it took to get here.
But I don't want to stop working or morning forward.
My goal is to get two more books out this year.

It goes back to the thoughts
"I can't do it again"
"I can't do it without tiny book course"
"I can't do it because creating a children's book is harder and different"
"I don't remember all the steps and how I even made that first one happen"
"I need a real job"

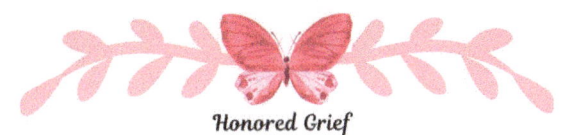

People wont support me like they did with the first book"
"The hype will be over now that I have already done it once"
"Who do I think I am? an author? just because I wrote 1 book?"
"I can't afford to make it happen again"
"Take your time, enjoy what's happening now first before jumping into more"

Then the more positive thoughts come in
"You have done this before; you can do it again"
"You have all the resources you need"
"You don't need to invest the same money you did before"
"You have a message the world needs to hear...or just 1 person, even if that 1 person is you"
"Listen to your intuition. Trust your calling"
"Do what makes you happy"
"Remember how good it feels"
"You can take all you learned to do things differently, you can learn more"
"You will always make mistakes, it's ok-that's your power"
"You have time"
"If not now, when?" why wait?

This first book is just one piece of me and my story. It was not even the full version of it.
I ended 2020 with "this is just book one, in 2021 there's more to come".

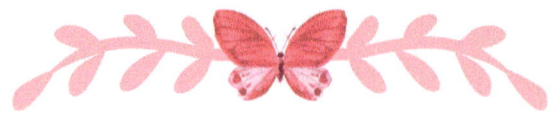

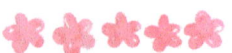

I feel that, I know that, I believe that.
Now, I must work on that. Because dreams take work.
And I am trying to hold on to all the good from this
experience to get me through.

Juan Ayala

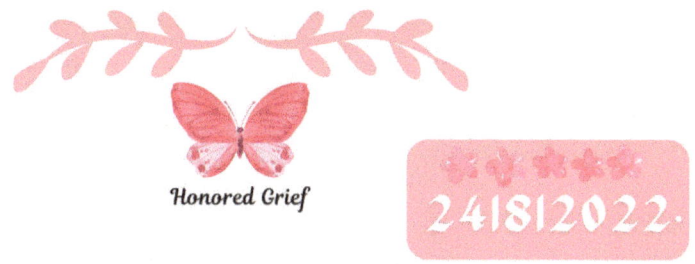

Honored Grief

241812022·

What does fulfillment mean to you?

Today it has looked and felt like many moments. Such as waking up before my morning alarm, and feeling rested and ready. Biking both shifts to work, feeling stronger and stronger day by day. Being in the fresh air. Knowing I have a job I enjoy that gets me on my bike.

Surrendered healing meetings. Writing letters to girls I have never met but knowing it will reach someone. My husband bringing me a delicious lunch. Making dinner at home. that everyone enjoys. Showering, washing my hair, shaving. Alone.

Cousins coming over from across the street to spend time with leo. Tiny mat group, book night. Skills group, mindfulness and meditation practice.
Making future credit card payments, setting dates - knowing payday is coming. My great niece's birthday. 5 revised books making it here, loving what I see. reflecting on this journey

To me, fulfillment is many moments added up. It is living dreams and following my heart: being a mom, wife, teacher, coach, author. People I have met.
It is a delicious meal that makes you do a happy dance. It is "if I died tomorrow, would I be happy with the life I have lived" It is not, not having dreams or

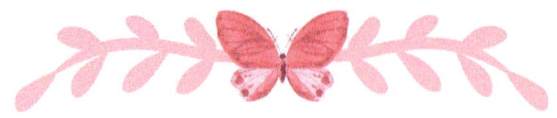

goals because I have so much more I want to do and live. But it is being at peace and feeling in alignment and so happy with where I am at, have been and am going.

It is a sense of being.

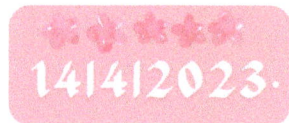

14|4|2023.

What are you being called to do?

I have been called since last year (and years before) to hold grief space (I started talking more about it last year)
And holding writing spaces

I was thinking of holding space for people to write a book
While I write my next
Kind of go through journey together
Maybe this summer

The details or when or how or all that not really known
But it's been on my heart.

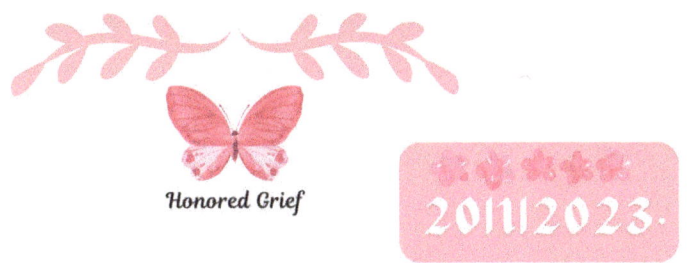

Honored Grief

20|11|2023·

Grief is the memories I have left
It is the good, the bad, everything in-between- all the things I can't forget.
Grief is more than just memories
memories, are more than just memories- they are everything.
They are all I have left.
All that is left of you. Of us.

Miss you always. love you forever.

Tomorrow will always be what tomorrow will be.
Nothing can change the date.
Nothing can take away what happened.
Nothing will bring you back. not in the way I mean.

Already our tomorrow plans have altered, due to someone trying to steal our car.
Already the day cannot be everything we wish it to be.

But it can still be. it can still be what we wish it to be.
We will still honor you.

Tomorrow will be what it's going to be. ....
and today, is today

I cannot be present for you right now.
In this present moment, all that is present for me is sadness, and I do not want to bring anyone else down.

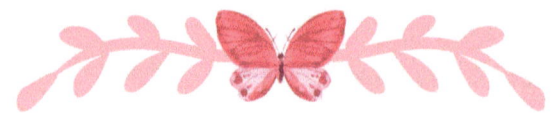

The moment I let it out and said I cannot be there for you. It hit me all that much harder, because I am accepting the truth. The truth that my dad's passing is still very hard on me.

I wasn't trying to ignore or avoid it, but the day has been ok up until now. and now I need to grieve.
The tears are flowing, they are crashing down
the baby comes in, and I need her to get out.
I do not want anyone around
Trying to make sense of why it is all hitting me right now.

I do not want to vision the future right now, knowing he is not in it
knowing right now I do not care to do anything else except be in this moment.
As I feel like I am in pieces of me
right now, this is what I need from me.

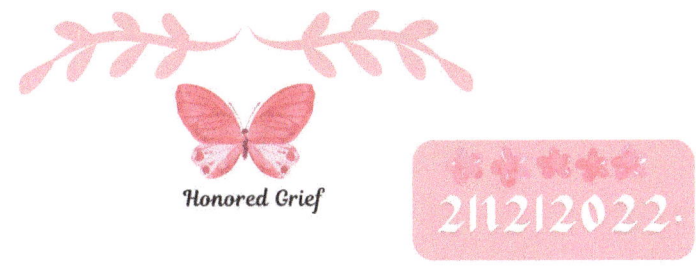

Honored Grief

2|12|2022·

All the grief I haven't grieved
Is where I'm at right now
It does not mean this workshop or time will heal or fix
or solve.
We do not need fixing.
We need time to feel our feelings.

How have I been making time for tears?

Realizing how desensitized I have become
Realizing how busy culture has me feeling rushed
Realizing how gratitude has become my crutch for
moving along
But not moving on
Turn on a song. Pictures. Write

Take time in the bathroom or shower or put a movie
for the kids or even find a sitter to sit alone.
Healing while writing
Is what's been real all along

Grief doesn't just go away
But can find a way to make peace, heal, partner
Gratitude is not a band aid or solution
It's a practice to shift mindset
Which leads to different actions and outcomes

How do you grieve?
What does it look like and mean?

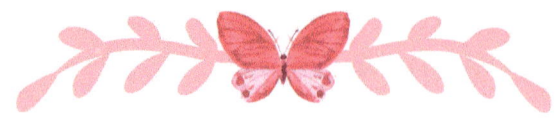

It can be journaling, sitting quiet, screaming, crying, music, dance,
Celebrating
Celebration of life

Because it's hard to be with the hard feelings
Because "they don't want us sad" but they deserve to be honored
Grief and Gratitude.

7112/2022.

All the grief I haven't grieved
(Reflecting with my feelings and thoughts)
might be my next workshop

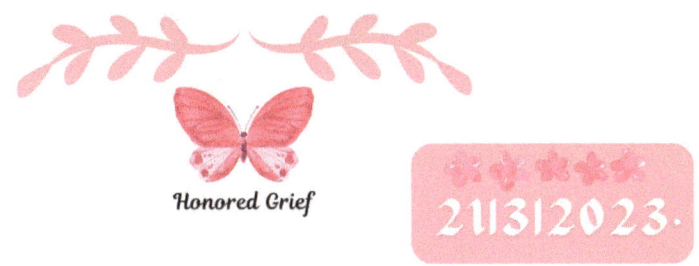

God knew I needed to see this
To Feel this. To Share this. Today.
A video of my dad's funeral popped up in my fb memories.
It was the song "hero" being sang by someone my dad cared for. A song I once sang at a school event that my dad attended. Facebook wouldn't let me share the video. So, I recorded with my phone and shared through there. Tears of course.

I just got off a call with my counselor, lots of conversation about feeling the feelings.
I am very logical and have somewhat detached from feeling emotions in a body scan type of way.
I have been moving quickly through and with life for the last year and a half. Not wanting to "back track" in areas I made "progress and change."

And now I am in so much physical pain, since November. It's been pretty consistent and constant.
It has been said and suggested, that the inflammation and pain may be tied to some emotional parts of me that I haven't fully allowed to be with.
I am all for feeling my feelings. But lately I have been in care taking and healing mode, that I have pushed some things to the side. Thinking I was ok.
Thinking I was doing right, with my past experiences and learnings and growth.

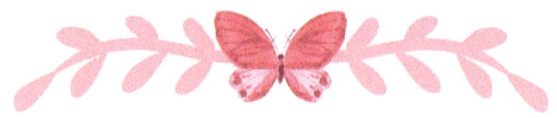

But there's some stuff there, it isn't even too deep in. I have known it, seen it, felt it- for so long.

I said it much of last year---there's so much grief I haven't grieved. Because the blessings were and have been just as big, if not bigger.

I think I need that time, more time-with the losses, the changes, the grief. And I keep working on it. But I know I need to spend more time in it and with it when it's present.

My dad's passing taught me....

- To take more videos of our mother's voices
- Ask hard questions like: what kind of burial do you want?
- That life insurance is so important
- Knowing your parents (loved ones) wishes feels significant
- Being ok with being ok was a lot harder than being ok with not being ok
- To be more present
- Next time...to look for/ask for/say yes to grief support/counseling/programs. for us and our kids

My dad's passing lead me to...

- Write books. Become an author.
- Get our moms books to write in, to leave behind for us and the grandkids

My dad's passing reminded me.....

- You can make things of people even while they are alive- like blankets and pillows and shirts. In their honor, not just in their memory.
- How gratitude saves me, over and over again.

My mothers-in-law's passing, so far-has taught me....

- That my dad's passing only prepared me so much
- That this grief journey is different in so many ways while similar
- That healing is continuous and so is the hurt
- How much inner work I have truly done before this

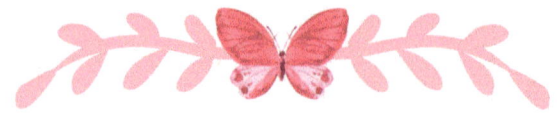

time came, during and after.

- For me, not being her "blood" feels different than being my dad's child. For me, it has made the grieving process different. My mind has held me back even when my emotions felt true and worthy. I still have so much "work" to do and things to learn.

My mother-in-law's passing lead me to....

- Questions I wish I knew to ask (like if she would leave each kid something of hers, even myself.)
- Realizing I thought my healing and journey with my dad was to help serve me for this journey. and it did. but also-there simply was stuff it could never prepare me for
- Speak up. for me, for my husband, for my kids. helped me speak up in conversations with them.
- New insights.
- Saving facebook words and posts, to create gifts for my loved ones.
- Honoring her and my dad in new ways

My mother-in-law's passing reminded me....

- How human I am
- How much I still did not know, about grief and how to prepare
- That not allowing your feelings to be felt physically, can lead to physical pains
- We can do healing together as a family and it is also important to have our own individual space.

Honored Grief

101712021

I met Estella Lopez and her family through my dad. Her mom Catrina was one of his good friends, she has been the person who does our taxes ever since my dad passed.

Estella is and does many things. I have admired her and been inspired by her. She has had an in-home childcare for a long time, she paints children's houses, she is a woman of GOD and faith.
In this video she is sharing about her grief and healing journey from losing her grandmother (catrina's mom) Catrina's mom actually sent me a card after my dad passed, I was so surprised. When this loss happened to the world, it included mine. I started sharing a couple of messages with estella and catrina. They did purchase "my book" as well.

While estella is talking...she shares about my book and I am just in "awe" jaw-dropping.
My reaction: Oh, my goodness can you feel my tears falling and my heart bursting of emotion.
Not because you are sharing "my book" (although thank you for that) but because of how it helped or served. I am blown away and know more that I am living in my purpose and this helped remind me.
I am still processing your words.

This whole video is so vulnerable and transparent and is medicine for so many. Thank you. So much love.

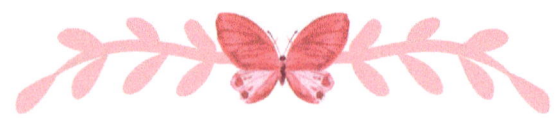

I found this video because I had read a post she made.
I had commented:
I feel like I was reading a book, one that many could benefit from.
Thank you for sharing your experience and honesty.
Rest In Peace to your grandmother ✨
And she said:

"I talked about your book in the middle of my last video posted and how it helped me through many of the steps I was taking at the time I bought two copies. Your book was a hand that held mine ...while I journeyed on some rough days. Juan Ayala was a one of a kind man and he would be so proud of you. You're helping many friend. ❤️"

So of course I wanted to watch and hear the video because just with those words shared....
I felt so much:
 "You have no idea what this means to me.
Thank you for sharing this with me.
Thank you for helping me move forward ❤️✨
My dad definitely put you all in my life for so many reasons, I am so thankful."

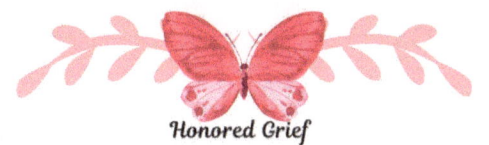

Honored Grief

25|06|2023.
Carolina
Velasquez

The grief I haven't grieved.
What does it mean to grieve?

By definition, it's deep sorrow - that caused by someone's death especially. The 7 stages can include: denial, anger, bargaining, depression, acceptance, hope and processing.

I have felt these feelings and stages at times in my life, where death of a person wasn't always the cause but the end of a relationship, the loss of something sentimental, even such things as moving or losing a job.

The grief I haven't grieved,
can mean so many things.

Maybe you have tapped into your grief here and there, allowed some uncontrollable tears.
allowed some tears to fall or thoughts to be present,
Maybe you dried them up as fast as they fell, maybe that quick cry was enough in that moment.
Maybe the thoughts came and went,

Often time grief doesn't just go away- it might take a break but it also might need some real attention.
Some real intention, time to be.

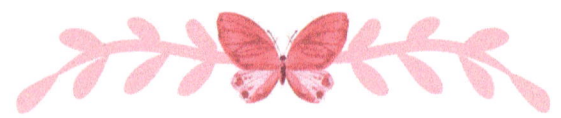

To be with yourself and all you are feeling.
I invite you to come as you are, however you wish to be. However you choose to share your journey.

When I say normalize
I don't mean desensitize.

Quite the opposite actually,
I want you to feel your feelings.

When I say lets normalize grief,
I mean lets take the time we need.

Lets be real with how we feel
lets allow ourselves to not be told how long it takes to heal.

Allow your truth to be true
allow life to slow down, to feel what you need to because it is the way through.

We may bandaid a feeling or situation for a moment but eventually we have to deal with it.

Wounds don't just heal
sometimes wounds are attached to the things we feel.

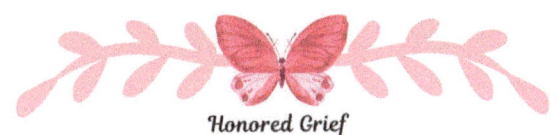

Honored Grief

Emotions do so much to our bodies
what we feel has the ability to effect us physically.

Our thoughts are powerful enough to create the actions we take
grief can rewire our brain, in ways.

There is power in coming as you are
the pieces of you are important to the pumping heart.

Your grieving heart is not what defines you
but anything will mean whatever we give meaning to.

I believe there is healing in feeling
even if the feeling isn't what we want to be feeling.

I am not saying to live in your grief
I am saying to spend some time instead of ignoring or masking the reality.

I do not hold space with the intention to cure of fix
anyone who grieves, knows- this is non-existent.

I have no answers anymore powerful than you
I am no expert, anymore than you and your truth.

I am a space holder
willing to share my story so that we can learn and grow together.

I am here to support you in grounding in your true self

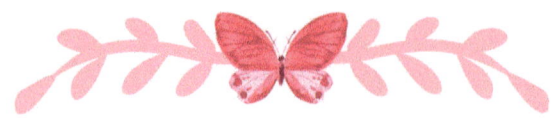

to support you in embracing you as a whole, even when the pieces feel like pieces and nothing else.

16|2|2023.

I keep grasping for happiness
Going to what works
But nothing is working
Grief...grieving

Honored Grief

#9popupoetry

You get scared.
To make an event and have the thought people might not be there.
People show interest and that is amazing in itself
but interest isn't an investment in the event itself.
People start to sign up
it's getting real, I try not to think of anything too much.
Because it's easy to assume, all that can go wrong
was I clear in what's to be expected? Your mind will make up so many reasons why people might of.

I don't have to think too much, there's still time until the day of
Then, it's the day before and you look to see how many people actually paid and signed up.
No number of expectations. Just wanting to kind of know the information for preparation.
But I can't really prepare what is meant to flow
There's no real script for holding space to be together-
to be real and know how it will go.

So many thoughts, ideas and heart felt directions
but no clear "how to" and there is time limitation.
I am not the teacher or leader
I just want to be the space holder.
The one that shows up real and transparent.
In hopes others will appreciate that and feel comfortable to do the same, even in silence

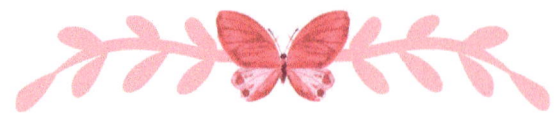

I wont really know why God keeps calling me to do this. I don't know, that i will know-even after i do this. But i know the calling has been for years
and i am answering the call now, even with the unknowns- even with the fears.

Writing my next book...
Today's tasks include- going through saved messages to type onto the computer.
Just type them and erase from phone.

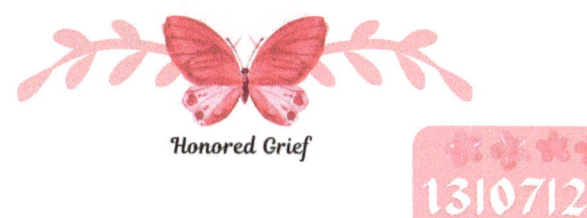

I hour until flow time.

Because I almost said "go time" but I am in no rush,
And I am aiming for faith and flow.

At this point I started to get nervous.

Lets be real, yesterday when I heard 15 people were signed up.

And now at 20 people.

Thoughts are flowing in:
*What are people expecting?
I can't know and don't need to know. How crazy would that make me, to know/
*I have no "plan"---just what's in my heart.
some notes on a paper that say things like : remember to breathe, to tell them to breathe, explain the title and why you are here.
Use journal prompts in the meditation.
and follow your heart.

----I started to get scared and looked up a meditation.
One about body scans.
because I started telling myself and feeling like "I need to do what's been done before"
"I need to do what I have seen work"
"who am I to create my own meditation"
But, using what's been made -didn't feel right, at all.
not because it wasn't mine.
but because it wasn't what my heart was telling me to do.

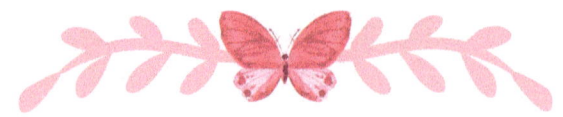

My heart didn't have a plan or script but it had a few thoughts and flow.
I ended up leaning into my heart.
ever since talking to heidi on the ferry weeks ago.
I knew I wanted to be authentic.
I knew I didn't know all the exacts, but that I was feeling like I needed to create my own-in order to hold the intention for the space and to see what could become.

The idea to ground in what's real, to make time to feel, to come as you are and then to journal right after and let the words flow. then to share out loud if wanted.
I had the fear of doing what "hasn't been done" of doing "what's new for me" fear of the unknowns.
Fear of judgement? maybe? but more so fear of expectations of me and the space. I just want it to be our space. I want to just "be me" and if what happens here is not for everybody or anybody-then that's ok.

But as long as I am authentic, those who are meant to be or wanting to be here now and, in the future, - then they will be.
I am holding that with me. That GOD has a plan for me. even if I can't see what that is.

Let's do this.....

"Seriously, thank you. I feel like our kids could benefit from it too" referring to the space held tonight. "The Grief I Haven't Grieved".

"Thank you for holding the space! Spirit definitely channeled through you bc it felt so natural and flowed so beautifully. I felt held and safe to feel thank u thank u thank u"

"Awesome job so proud of you."

"You. are. outstanding. inspiring. wow"

"That was amazing, thank you for giving me the chance to connect with my own grief. I appreciate you and your journey."

"It was like spirit took over your body. You are in your purpose, it just flowed."

And when it was over...I cried...

"GOD, I did it."

And so much gratitude for all who showed up and my Team".

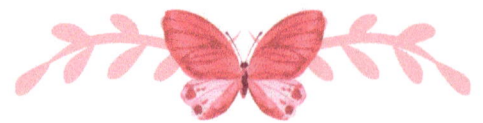

14|07|2023·
Carolina
Velasquez

Shared with your friends

It's going to take me some time to process yesterday. The time leading up to, during and moments after. It's the morning after and I am still processing...

Thank you to everyone who attended "The grief I haven't grieved." I had mentioned that this has been a calling for the last couple of years now and I wasn't exactly sure why but I just knew the call continued calling- so I decided to finally really answer.

For me this experience has come in layers. From naming it to claiming it and to doing it. From people showing interest, to people signing up- even on the day of! Felt like confirmation that this is something "needed" and not just for myself.

When people showed up, shared in chat or off mute, on screen or off, with emojis or simply were just present--all of it was deeply appreciated and matters to me.

The gratitude's at the end and the comments of what the space meant for people- means so much to my heart and my purpose.

I am deeply thankful for you all and wanted to be able to share my gratitude.

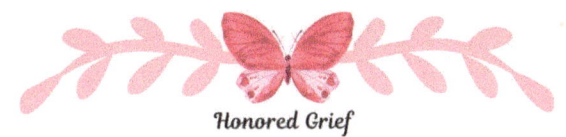

Honored Grief

I know in my heart , I will hold space again.
Space for grief, to come as you are, for journaling, for community and for gratitude.

I don't know when or what changes will be made, but I do know- yesterday showed me a bit of why I am being called.

Yesterday showed me people would like more.
more space for themselves, to just give themselves this time they did or didn't know they needed.
this time that can feel vulnerable and heavy while also feel like a sense of healing.
this time that is, self-care.

thank you to any friend, family, new face-who took a chance on me. on trusting me to hold space even if you didn't know what to expect. even if you were hesitant to come. even if you just came for me but left with so much more.
mutually connected through grief but it's so much more than that because the layers are so many.
journal prompts can lead to so many places and conversations.

I love that this time, was just for coming as you are. being seen, held and honoring who/what we are grieving by naming them.

Thank you Jasmin and Brie, for the grounding sanctuary.

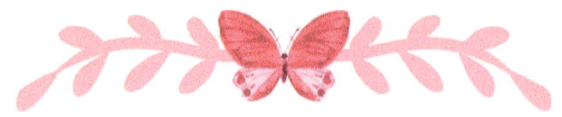

For the space to allow me to be me and flow through and yet I felt held and supported.

Thank you for making me not just feel like, but to know- I am not alone and that although I can do anything on my own- I don't have to.
Being able to do this with yall, was a big part of why I finally answered the call.
It took away some of the scary parts of unknowns.
Community is a big part of my why, my values.
And ever since we had been a team, I feel like that path has continued. even if it looks differently.

Love yall.

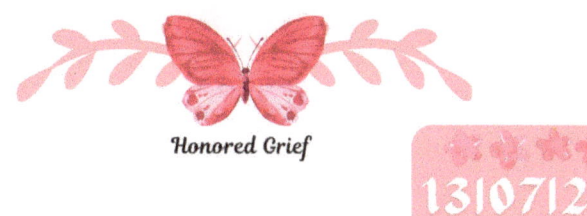

Honored Grief

I have been getting a lot of requests and asks:

- How often do you hold space at the grounding sanctuary?
- When will you be holding space for grief again?
- When is your next event?
- Would you be willing to hold space within my business?

Last month I finally held space for "The Grief I Haven't Grieved".

It had been years of having the calling and I finally said yes. I always knew I would. I always saw it as something I would do-

But for some reason not wanting to do "On My Own" not yet

I did it.

Learned so much. About me. About grief. About community. About the grounding sanctuary. About following my heart. About answering the call. About entrepreneurship. and more.

Honestly, still learning and processing.

I knew that day, and even before if I am being honest- that this wouldn't be a "one and done" thing

and, that is how it felt after that day.

I did it.

But it still felt "not done"

Like this would be, every so often

How often? I am not sure.

Because grief has no end.

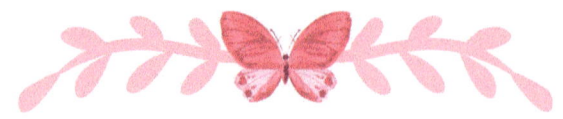

It's more like learning to live with
Well, yesterday I signed up to hold space again in September.....
I don't want the same title
I don't want anyone who joined to have exact expectations because honestly, that day was held from the heart.

No real plans, some rhythm but mostly just flow
and the next time I do this, I don't want to compare
not me to anyone else, even myself. It may look different---we may not ground in meditation
The intention will be the same, to be with our grief
To come as you are
To make it accessible
To have time for you, for journaling, time

I see myself holding this space
But there is so much to explore when it comes to grief and journaling and being that this can look so many ways. So, all I ask and offer is an invitation to come if you feel at all called.
to come as you are
To be open minded with no solid expectations of how the space will be--- because we will flow, we will ground, have time to slow down,
Time to feel whats real
Time to be with what is
Time to reflect (journal, think, be) and
Time to connect, all in community.
To share, to be heard, to be seen ---or not.

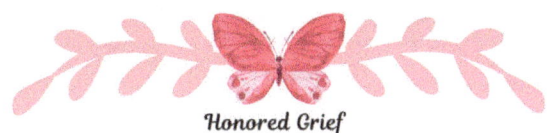

Honored Grief

To listen, to chat, to be together---however feels right for you in the space.

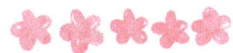

12/10/2023·

The grief
I haven't grieved
Is piling up
Inside of me

23/10/2023·

Come as you are,
For the grief you haven't grieved
The grief that hasn't been given permission to grieve because she wasn't "my mom" I put me to the side to be there for your grief.
Telling myself I cant compare
I know what it's like to lose a parent so I have to be fair. The part about my part in this is that you all as her children made me feel less important. Me watching everyone take dibs at belongings the day she passed
While my husband wasn't even thought of, while he was thought of last. The one thing I wanted was claimed.

I had to let it be ok.
I have to speak up for my children
Whether they ask or not

129

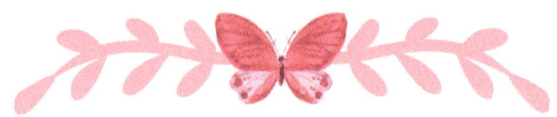

I'm thinking of their future- knowing how it feels to have loss. You as my husband, their dad. you need to speak up for us too.

We matter too, we lost her too.
I wish I thought of asking her for a keepsake before she was no longer here.

I wish I was thought of without having to ask, then we wouldn't be in this situation here.
I'm just the daughter-in-law but I felt like I was more, when she was here and now it's gone.

23|2|2023.

I don't share this to make anyone feel bad, that isn't my intention. My intention is to just be real with how I feel.

26|2|2023.

Sometimes we tone down or turn off our grief.

- Not wanting to take away from others
- Not feeling worthy enough to be in such grief.
- When it can't possibly compare to what others in the same circle are feeling.
- Feeling like we don't have the time
- Feeling like we need to be there for others more than ourselves
- Feeling like it's easier to be there for others than ourselves
- Sometimes we are numb to the loss
- Sometimes we don't want to face the reality the feelings and thoughts that arise

2|3|2023.

✨Daughter-in-law, not daughter.
A part of that has kept me from allowing my grief. 🙏
Unwilling to lose myself the way I did with my dad. 🪦
While also aware I am a different version of me, with this grief.

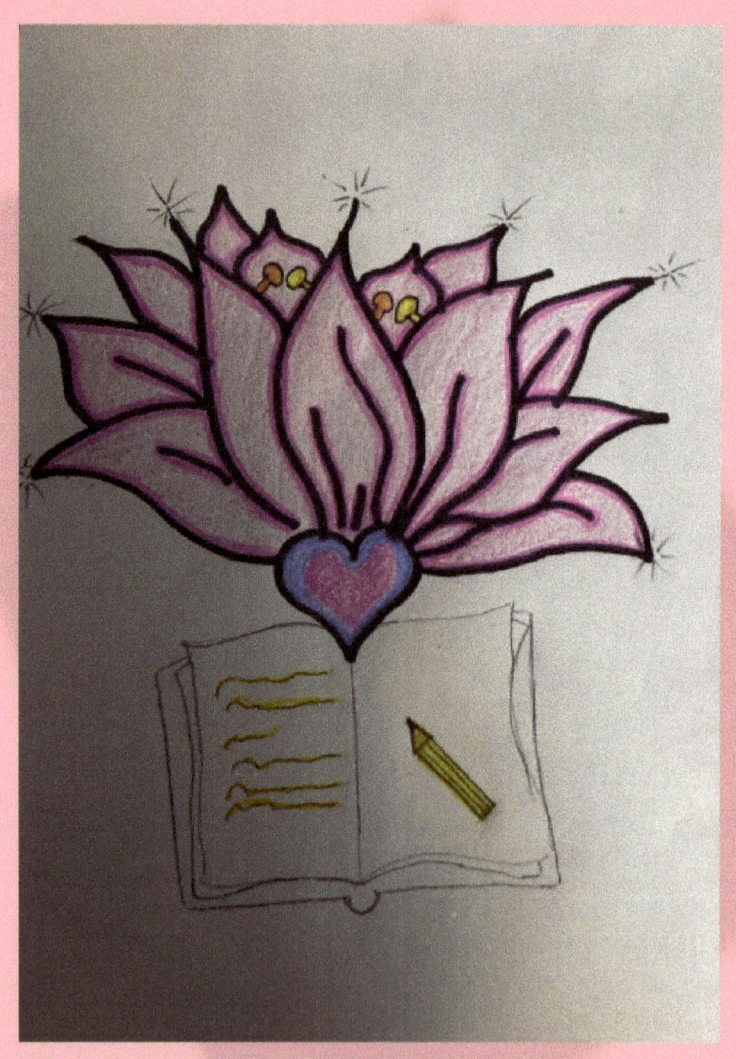

Chapter

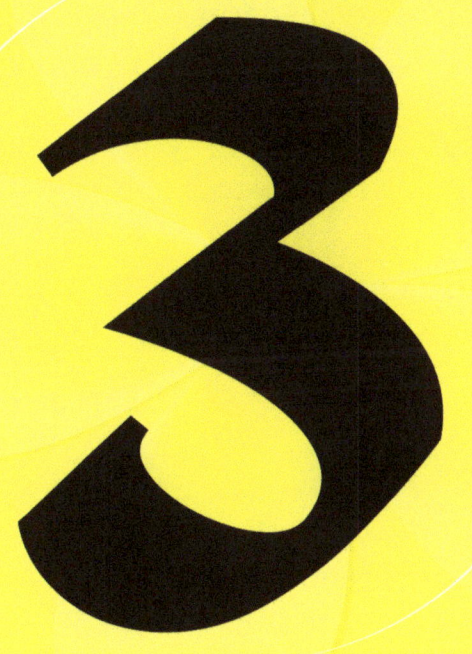

3

Healing While Writing

> Everything in my life, is my story and has created my journey. It is my brand. My truth is my marketing. I am my business.

> Turn your gifts into profit. Take your knowledge and create. Build yourself. Follow your heart.

> Today, grief made time for me. And in return,
> I made time to be with grief. To be with love,
> in love and present- while reflecting on the
> past (while being here, right now)

> What if, you meet yourself where you are?
> Surround yourself with people who support
> your mental health, your joy, your choice to
> choose, your health and your truth.

"
Your grief might take a break, It also might need some real attention and intention. Balance for me is about grounding, grounding by allowing my true self to be and embracing me as a whole. We are whole, all of our layers- it all connects. (mind, body and soul)
"

"
You are enough, as you are.
"

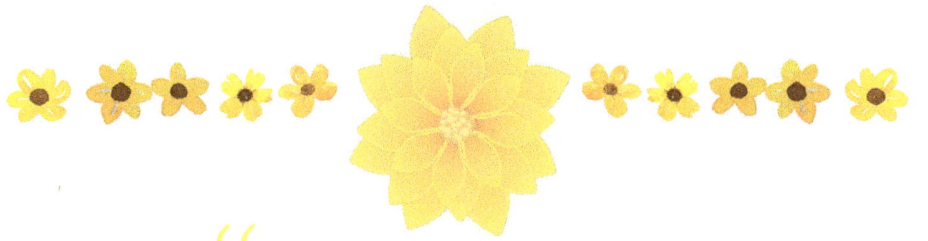

> Grief can "hit" you in ways and at times you least expect it. Sometimes it never feels like the right moment, time, or place.
> There's often not enough permission, or space to be with it.
> But what if there was?

> When the stress, fears and chaos are present. It is enough to trigger sickness, illness, pain and more. You can feel what is real and reframe still. Healing and medicine come in many forms.

> "
> Maybe you have tapped into your grief here
> and there. Allowed some uncontrollable
> tears to fall and dried them up as fast as
> they fell. Maybe that quick cry was enough.
> Maybe some overwhelming thoughts flood
> your mind- bringing up anger, sorrow, guilt,
> or shame. Often with grief, it does not just go
> away. Not forever.
> "

> "
> Grieve as you feel called.
> Be in community, listen, share.
> Navigating grief looks different for everyone.
> "

> If you can write a facebook post, You can write a book. (Or, a card deck.)
> If I can do it, anyone can. You can turn your grief into something "more".
> You can share your experiences and help heal the world.

> If you are being called to create.
> The "how" is not what matters most.
> know your why. Your heart.

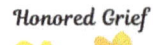

> (Just ask Google:
> Expressive writing can result in a
> reduction in stress, anxiety, and
> depression; improve our sleep and
> performance; and bring us greater
> focus and clarity).

> Grief really hits you in unexpected
> ways. I feel wrong for how I feel. I
> feel upset that my hurt is affecting
> how I treat others and how they
> feel. I feel upset that I can't get past
> my hurt quickly.

> I am also accepting it as it comes, as it is. I do not want to pretend it is what it isn't. This is my journey, and I am allowing it.

> I knew when you left, life would be different. I just didn't know; how different it would make me.

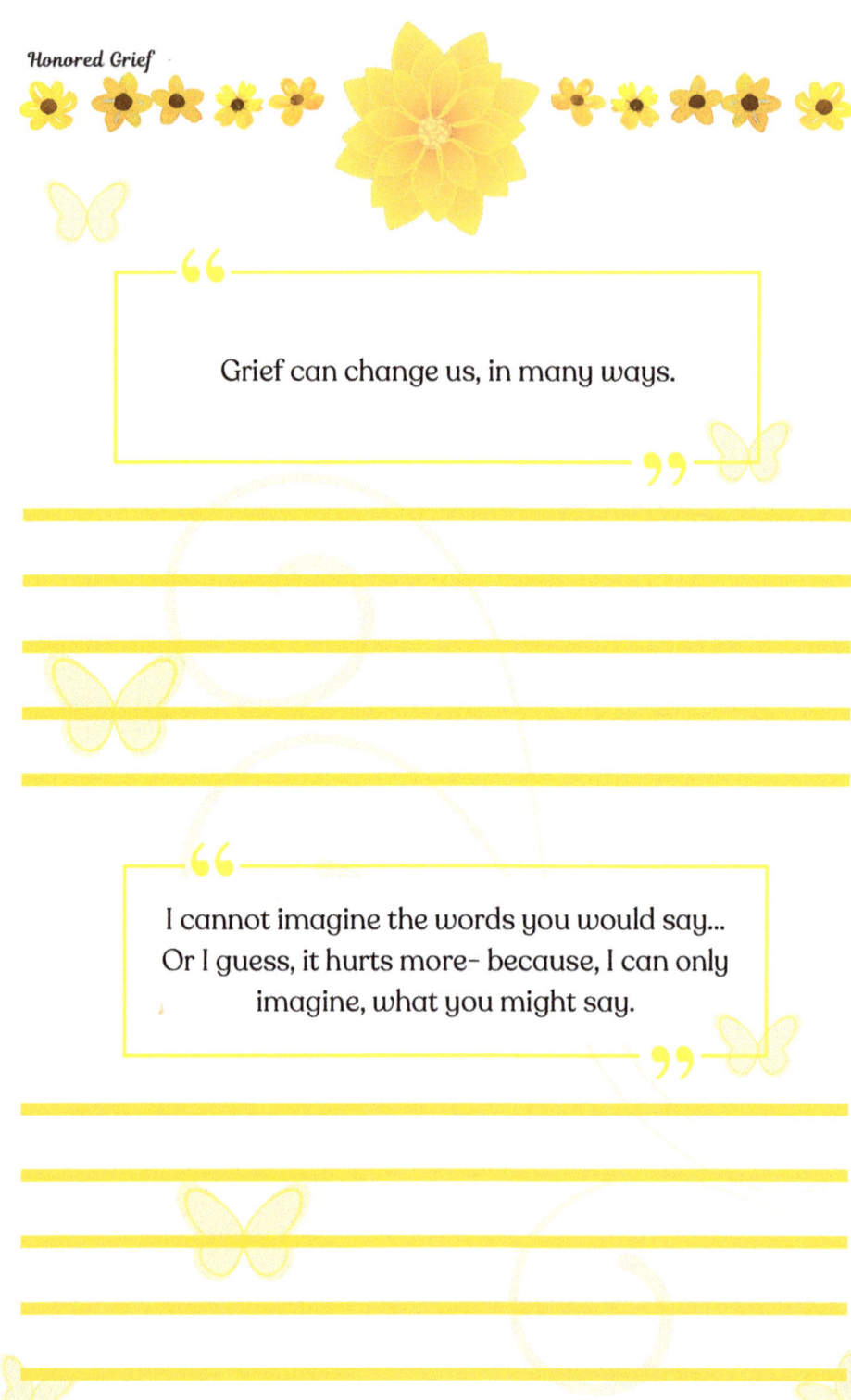

> Grief can change us, in many ways.

> I cannot imagine the words you would say...
> Or I guess, it hurts more- because, I can only
> imagine, what you might say.

> Share your truth, it may help others feel brave enough to accept their true feelings and thoughts- when it comes to grief.

> Honor them, while they are here. And when they are gone. You are allowed to be intentional with all experiences.

> All your feelings when grieving and healing are valid.

> Know that: it is ok, to not be ok.
> And, it is ok. To be ok.

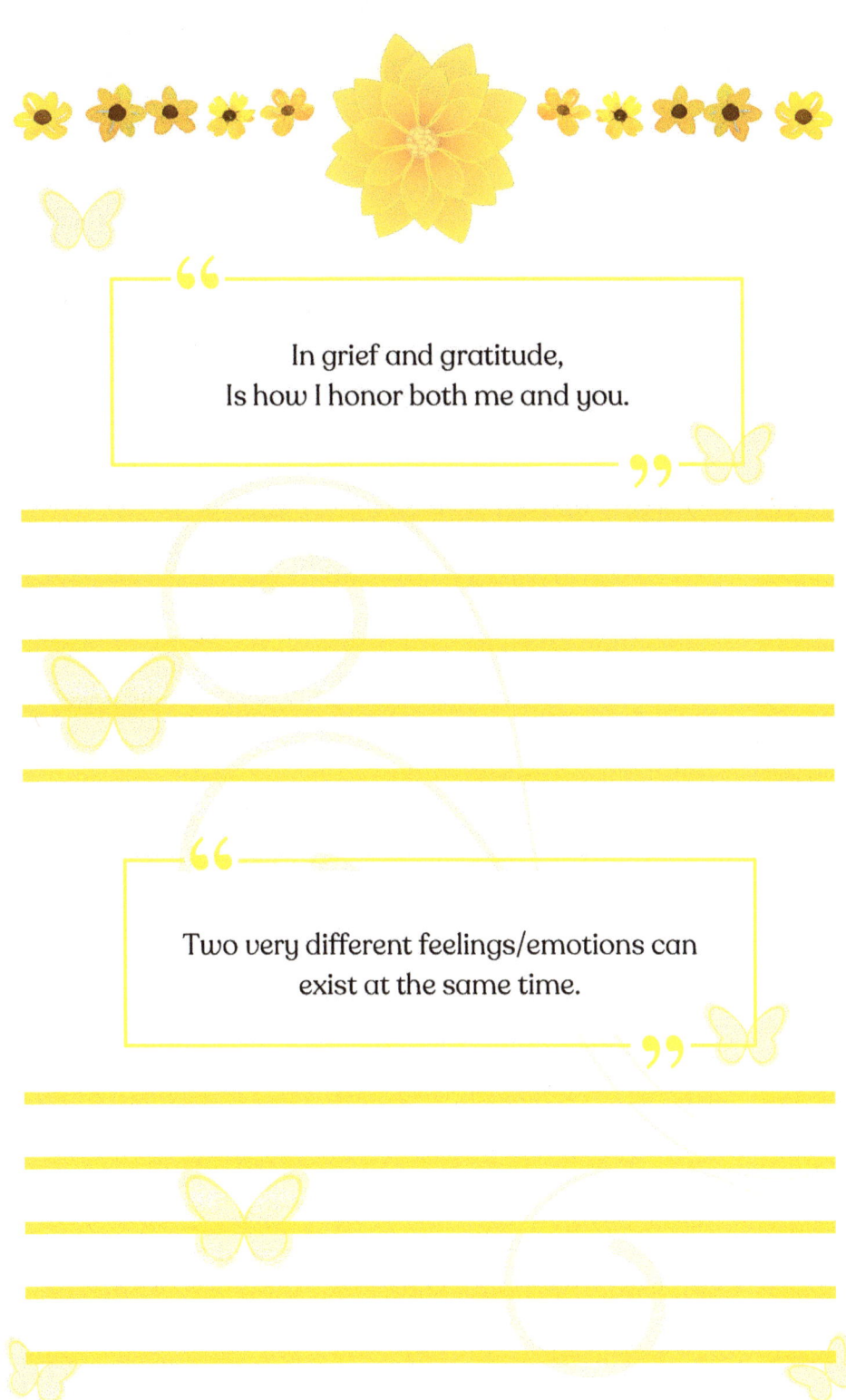

> In grief and gratitude,
> Is how I honor both me and you.

> Two very different feelings/emotions can
> exist at the same time.

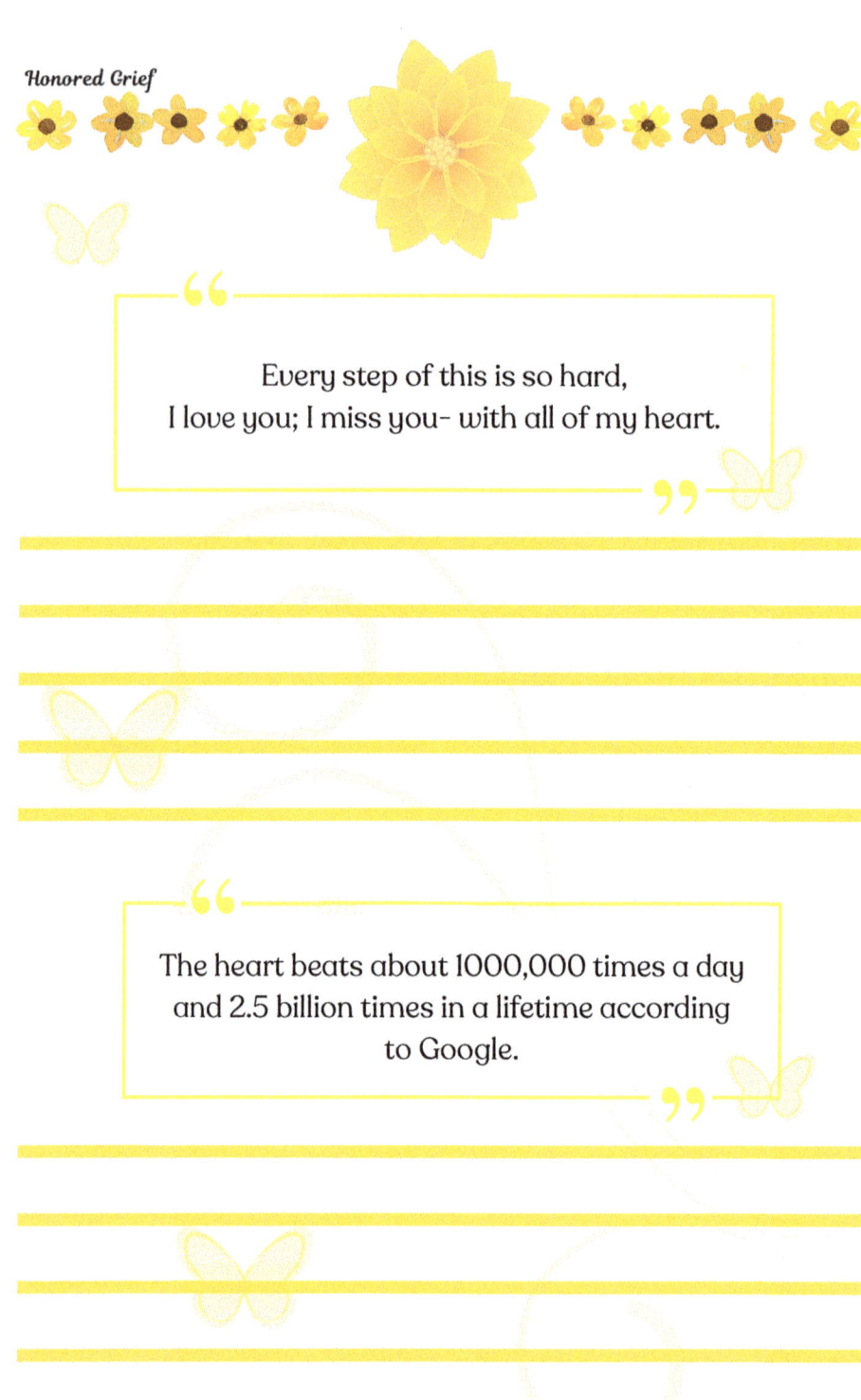

> Every step of this is so hard,
> I love you; I miss you- with all of my heart.

> The heart beats about 1000,000 times a day
> and 2.5 billion times in a lifetime according
> to Google.

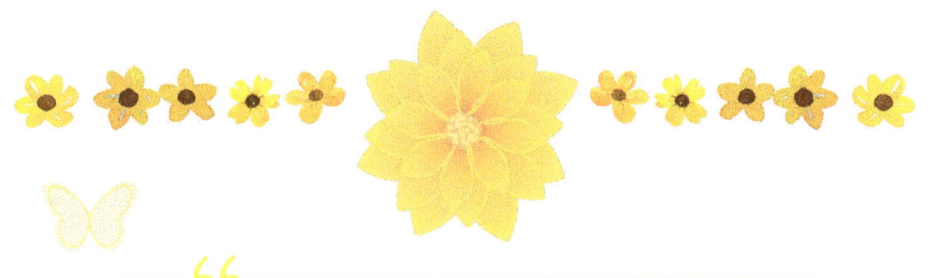

> Ignoring the truth,
> Does not make it not true.

> Its ok to heal.
> That does not mean that love is gone.
> Or that feeling "better" is wrong.

> "
> There is no right or wrong on your journey.
> Invitation to give yourself grace and space
> to feel what's real.
> "

> "
> It is ok to feel what you feel.
> It is ok to feel ok.
> "

> Say their names. Write their names.
> It is ok to miss who or what is "gone."

> What name would you give your grief?

> Sometimes when you are in your grief,
> It can feel like you start to lose people who
> are still physically here.

> Grief and grieving do not just become
> present when a death occurs.

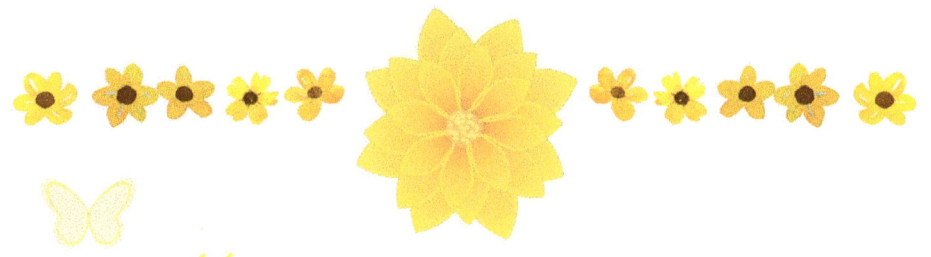

> You are whole, even when in grief.
> Even when you feel "broken"

> Normalize grief.
> Not desensitize.
> Normalize.
> That it is different to and for all.

> And that you are deserving, of your time, your truth. You have the permission, to grieve, to be. To not rush or be on anyone else's timeline.

> Celebration.
> Sometimes those tears fall easiest when the success comes. An accomplishment or a feel-good moment.

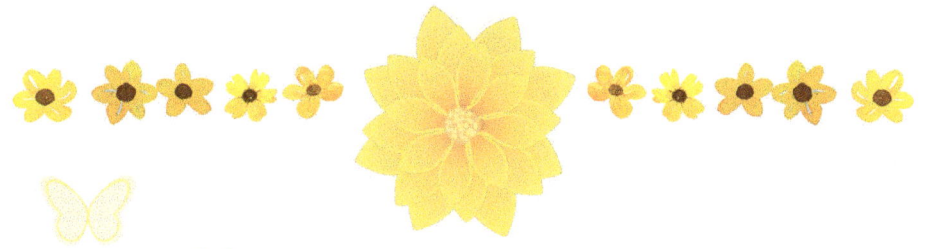

> Take time to be in it,
> In the moment. You deserve it.
> (Friendly reminder/permission: it is ok to feel
> good, even in grief.)

> This journey of grief.
> Is always ending and beginning again.

> It is more of a partnership, not something that has an end date. It's more of a relationship, that comes with ups and downs.

> Grief can show up in many ways:
> Constipation, tears, anger, sadness, memories, inflammation, back pain, anxiety, trouble sleeping, depression, nausea, fear, sickness, isolation
> What is your truth?

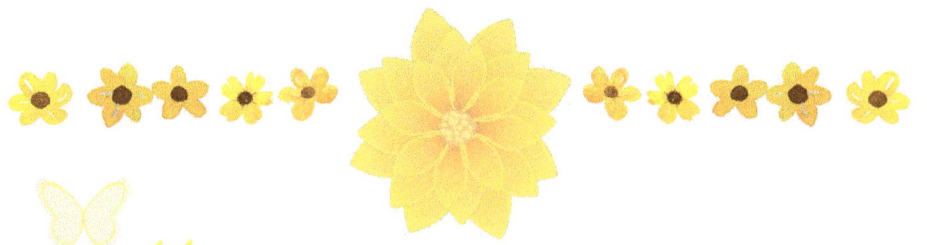

> Healing in grief can look like many things:
> Yoga, writing, reflecting, tears, going for a walk,
> prayer, going out into nature, talking, feeling your
> feelings, meditation
> What is true for you?

> Come as you are,
> For the grief you have not grieved.

"

Make time for your grief.

"

"

Grief and celebration can co-exist.
They do. With or without permission.
I have learned, that permission part – can
make a big difference.

"

> I wish it was that easy...
> So, I am going to let it be. Let it flow. Let me be
> me. Partnering with fear by holding hands but
> not giving it the power to stop what's trying to be.

> We are always healing. You don't have to be
> in tremendous pain or undeniable grief or
> severe depression or physically wounded–
> To be required or deserving or in need of
> healing. You are deserving, always.

> The stages of grief are said to be Denial: refusing to accept the reality of the loss. Anger: feeling resentment, rage, or blame towards oneself or others. Bargaining: trying to negotiate or postpone the loss or its consequences. Depression: feeling sadness, hopelessness, or despair. Acceptance: coming to terms with the loss and moving on.

> If you could title your grief with a movie or song, What would it be called?
> (This can change on any given day, at any moment. Feel free to come back to any question and see how it resonates at different times.)

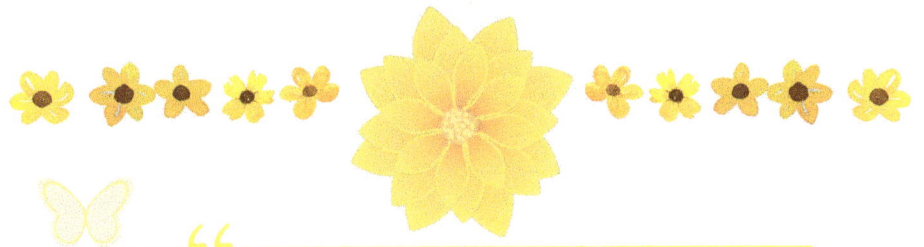

> If the person who died knew what you were feeling (anger, sadness, gratitude, fill in the blank). What might they say to you?
> How might they care for you?

> (It is ok for you to love yourself the way you love others.)
> Have you ever heard the saying "pain is love"?
> What does that statement mean to you?
> Do you agree or disagree? Why?

> How do you honor those who have died?
> How do you honor people/ situations/
> sentimental items you care about?

> Ask yourself this:
> What lessons has grief taught me?

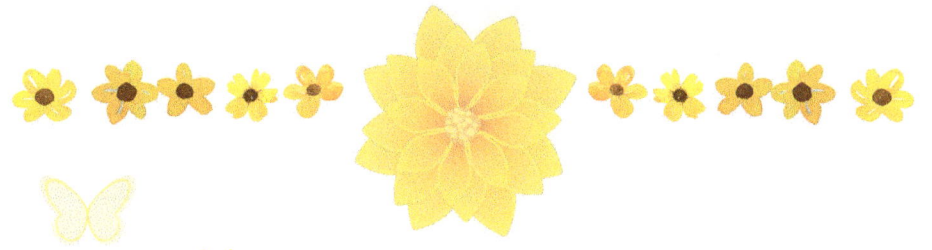

> How do you store your grief?
> (Feel free to: free write. Let the pen flow with
> whatever comes to mind.)

> What are you grateful for?
> Yes, right now. Anything. Allow it to flow.
> (memories, life, pictures, faith, ...what is true
> for you?)

> What left? What is left?
> (Please do what you feel is needed to take
> care of you. Cry, drink water or tea, breathe,
> light a candle...)

> What are the clear messages coming
> through to you?
> (From your body, ancestors, spirit, mind,
> emotions?)

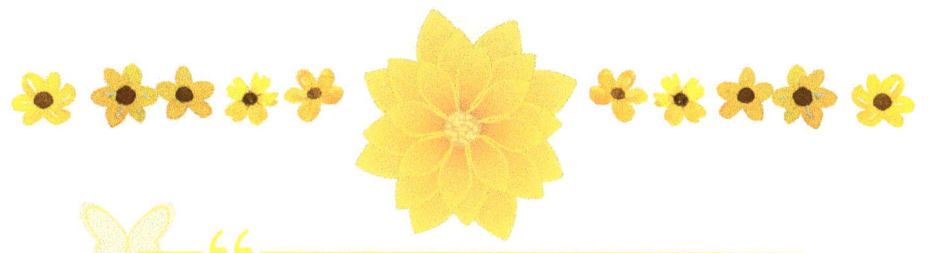

> If you gave your grief a voice, what would it sound like? What would it look like?
> (invitation to draw)

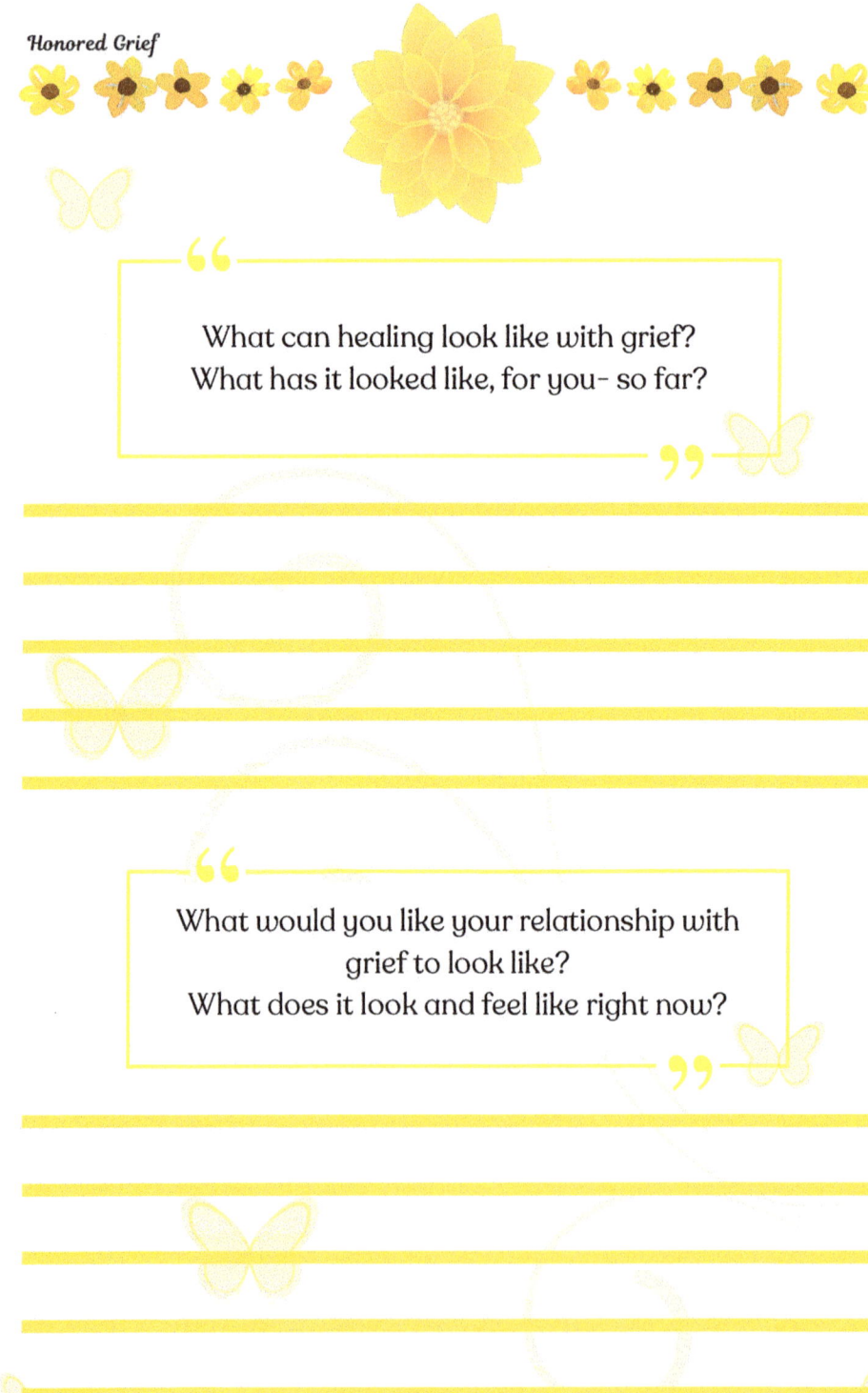

> What can healing look like with grief?
> What has it looked like, for you- so far?

> What would you like your relationship with
> grief to look like?
> What does it look and feel like right now?

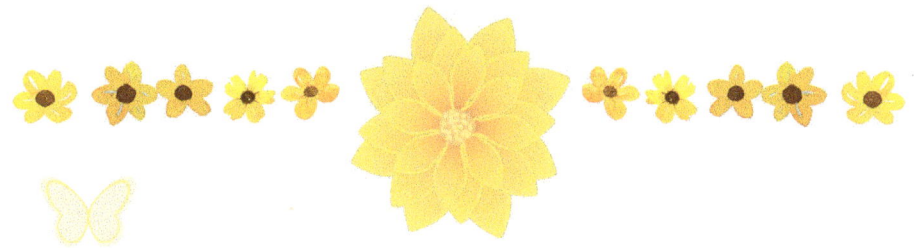

> What permission are you seeking,
> To grieve to the extent that feels needed for
> you? What would it look like, for you to
> grieve fully?

> How does grief show up in your life? In your
> body?

> **"**
>
> What does your grief want you to know?
> (Reminder to breathe. Inhale, exhale)
>
> **"**

> **"**
>
> What is your pain telling you?
> (ask yourself: what does my pain want me to
> know?) Maybe you want to journal, record a
> voice memo, just think to yourself...
>
> **"**

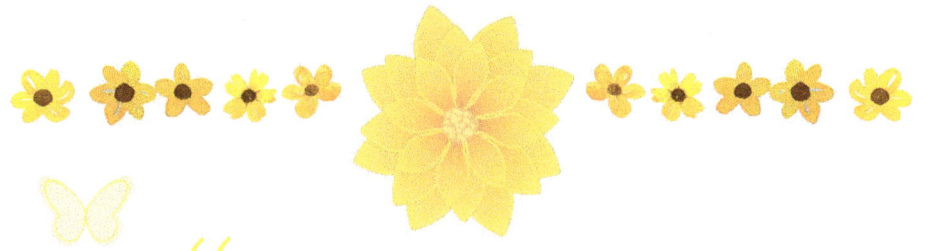

> What is grief? What does it mean to you?
> What has it meant to you, so far?
> (In the mood for poetry and writing.
> And feeling the feelings)

> If gratitude was a menu, what would be on it?
> If grief was a menu, what would be on it?

> You are not a failure because it didn't go the
> way you hoped. Sometimes the path comes
> with change, give yourself grace.

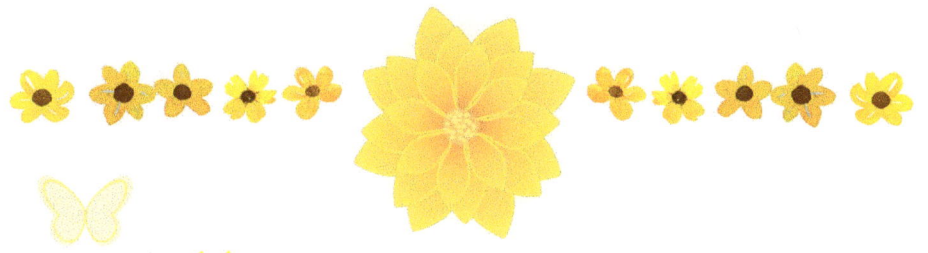

> If you knew you were supported and could not get hurt doing it, what would you leap into?

> How can you maximize your mindset today?

> "
> What can you teach others because of your
> own experiences, stories, learnings- on this
> journey of grief and healing?
> (what 5 things can you share?)
> "

> "
> What grief have you not yet grieved?
> (death, loss, pain... relationships, situations...)
> "

> When it comes to your grief, what is your intention when feeling it? What is your intention when you do not allow yourself to feel it? (anytime and as many times as you feel called...ask yourself "what is my intention?")

"
What helps you feel connected, to your loved ones?
To your grief? To your heart? (Everything is an invitation/example/idea...some things that may support you when journaling or reflecting: something to write with/on, items that bring you comfort peace inspiration, a private space, water, or tea to drink...)
"

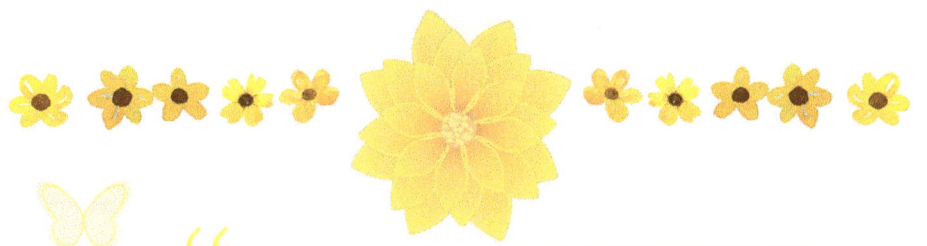

> What is the story on your heart?
> Invitation to take a deep breathe (in and out)
> and let your pen flow
> What story wants to be told?

> Finding peace through
> all the moving pieces.

> What meaning are you giving the word
> "goodbye."
> Are you in charge of your reality?
> What can you have control over?

> I use to be ok at goodbyes- I accepted reality
> I use to be ok with knowing death happens in
> life, until it took you from me.

> How powerful is your grief?
> How has it changed you?
> What has it shifted for you?

> If words could make it all ok, what would
> you say? (what would you like to hear, if it
> could change the way you feel)

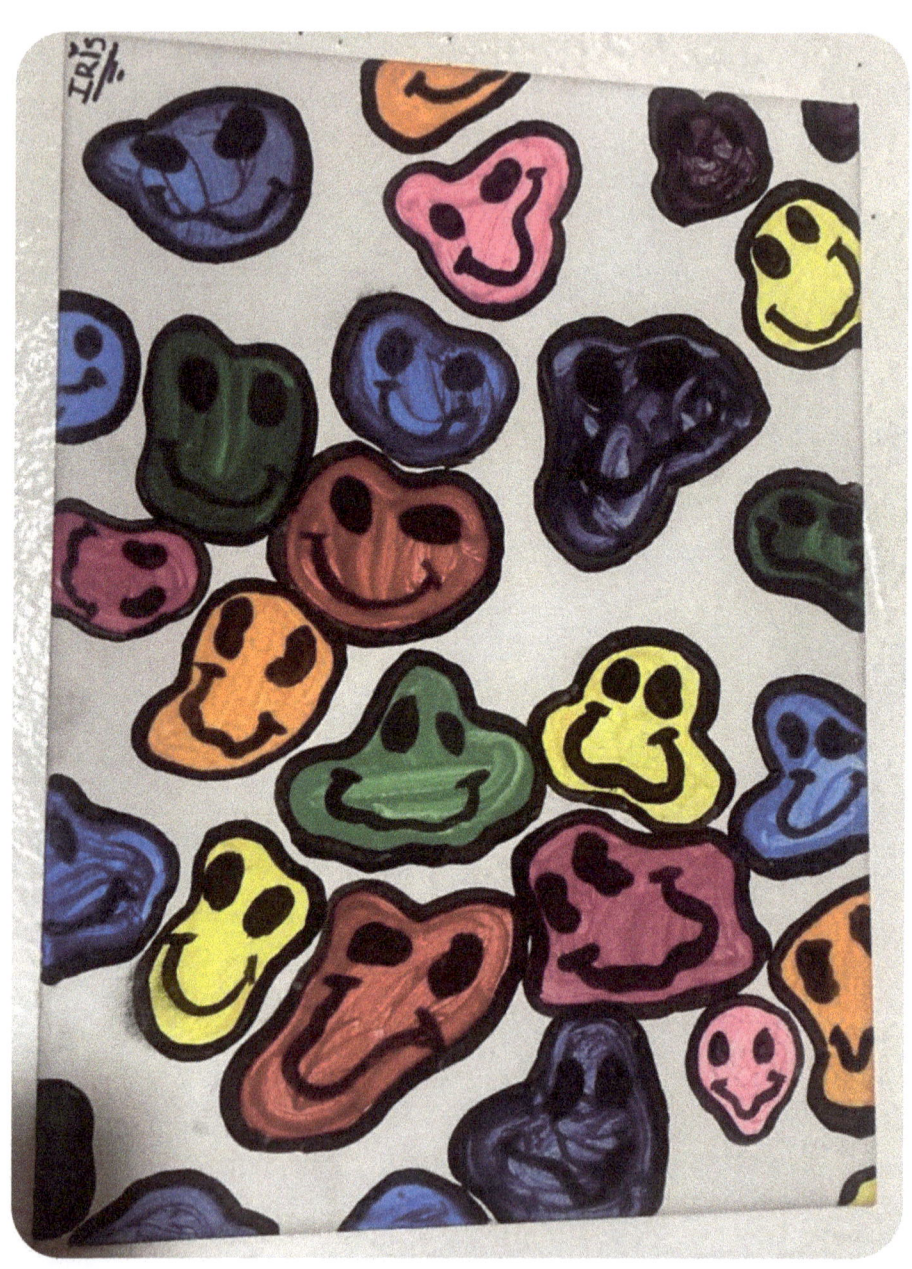

176

Thank you for sharing your truth and journey while grieving. Our time together was very meaningful and powerful.

I enjoyed hosting this interview and your book Healing While Hurting. Your words are needed especially during a time when many people have lost loved ones and are still coping with grief. See our conversation below.

Here are some tips Lena Ayala-Velasquez uses to deal with grief and self care:

1. Check in with yourself
2. Call off work
3. Eat your loved one's favorite meal
4. Give yourself grace
5. Give yourself permission to do what you need to do for YOU
6. Immerse yourself in enjoying pictures of your loved ones

From lena same day: It's Tuesday morning.
Sunday evening Natalie brought up the idea of us interviewing each other. We are both self-published authors.
we agreed, we would set a future date to do it.

Then this morning as I was thinking of my 1 year publish date tomorrow- I messaged her and said what about interview tomorrow?
We then decided today...which turned to right now....
We took 10minutes to put on earrings, makeup and hop on zoom,

during her lunch break.

It was that simple! two friends, two authors, two teachers, two people ----who are helping each other network. Helping each other grow. Helping each other learn and tell our stories.

We both asked each other questions that the other loved. No rehearsal, no time for re-dos. We can edit and snippet and share what we please. There's beauty in recordings. I still must learn how to do all of that. But, for now---here it is---in all of its realness and beauty.

I share this to say...

It is easy to support each other, to celebrate each other, to uplift each other, to network, to help each other grow. It did not take much time at all, to connect and to show up and to share.

I now get to add this to my list of what made 2021 great.

I got to interview someone. I got to be interviewed.

I put a little makeup on, embraced my natural curls and hair.

I got to talk about something thats hard for me, take deep breaths, smile and live in the moment. we embraced the moment, the unpolished realness and flowed with it.

I am so thankful .

Shout-out to Brooklynsfortune (I am wearing my new sweater) and it's so comfortable and I feel an extra sense of pride to wear something created by someone I used to go to school with/run track with. Jasmine

And shout-out to soulutionintuitivedesigns (jasmine)for the back

ground you created for surrendered healing that allows me to hop on zoom and hide my background life. With this beautiful background I am reminded of my best self, all that I am a part of now and the comfort the waves give me.

Gratitude

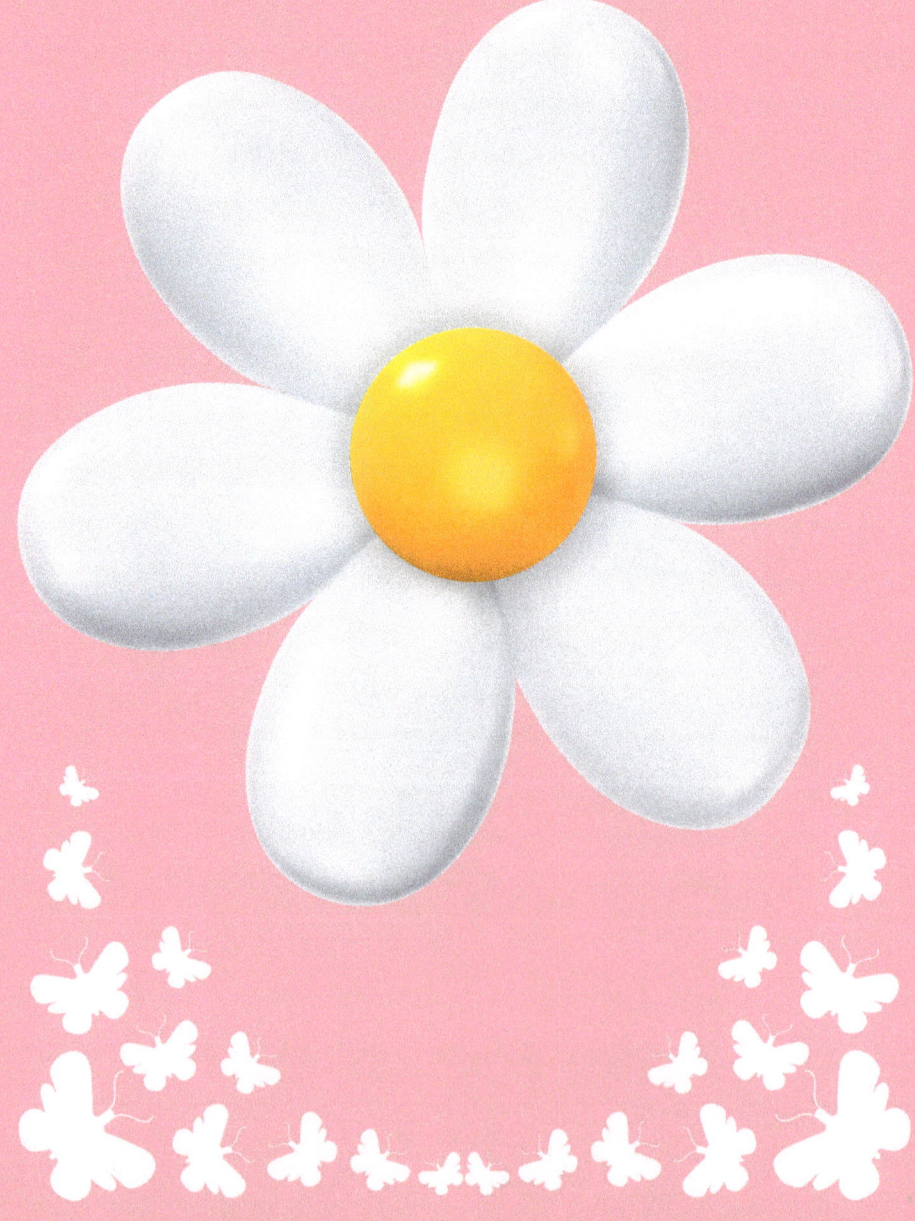

Thank you to GOD, for your love and never-ending support. For my faith and trust. For prayers. For tears held that no one will ever know about. For spirit. For intuition. For connection to ancestors. For gifts given.

Thank you to all who contributed in any way. For your vulnerability, your voice, your truth, your heart, your share.

Thank you to my mother-in-law, Martha. For your heart. For the way you were raised, for your beliefs, for your shared faith, for your honesty, for your inventions whether that be through art or cooking or healing. Thank you for the grandmother you are, the mother-in-law you are, the mother I witnessed. Thank you for your son, for your children that became my family and your family that became our family. Thank you for sharing memories, grief, love and life with me. Thank you for the times playing board games and watching movies. Thank you for all you did, to be able to be here with us -as long as you were.

Thank you to my father, for the man you are- for your heart, for the way you lived, for your changes when it came to addiction and a traumatic past. Thank you for your honesty, your protection, your humor, the grandfather you are, the father-in-law you are and the man you are. Thank you for the way you loved us. And continue to be here for us in spirit. Thank you to my mom, I am so grateful GOD has allowed you to still be here with us. Thank you for being here for me- even at 35!

Thank you for the grandmother you are, the only way you know how to be "real." Thank you for the person you are- you love unconditionally, you are very giving with what you have, you are funny without trying and you support us through whatever. Thank you to my husband and children.

Thank you for inspiring me-without trying. Thank you for allowing my truth to be. Thank you for choosing in on being a part of this book creation, thank you for sharing pieces of yourself with us. Thank you for jumping into this world with me. Thank you for being open-minded and for also setting the boundaries necessary for you.

Thank you to everyone who is in my life. For being a part of my journey, my healing, my grief. Thank you to me, to my heart, for answering inner calls, for following dreams, for my faith and my persistence and authenticity.

Thank you, for taking this life with all the ups and downs and being able to ground in gratitude and love. Thank you for allowing all parts of who you are to matter because they are all valuable and real. Thank you for being you.

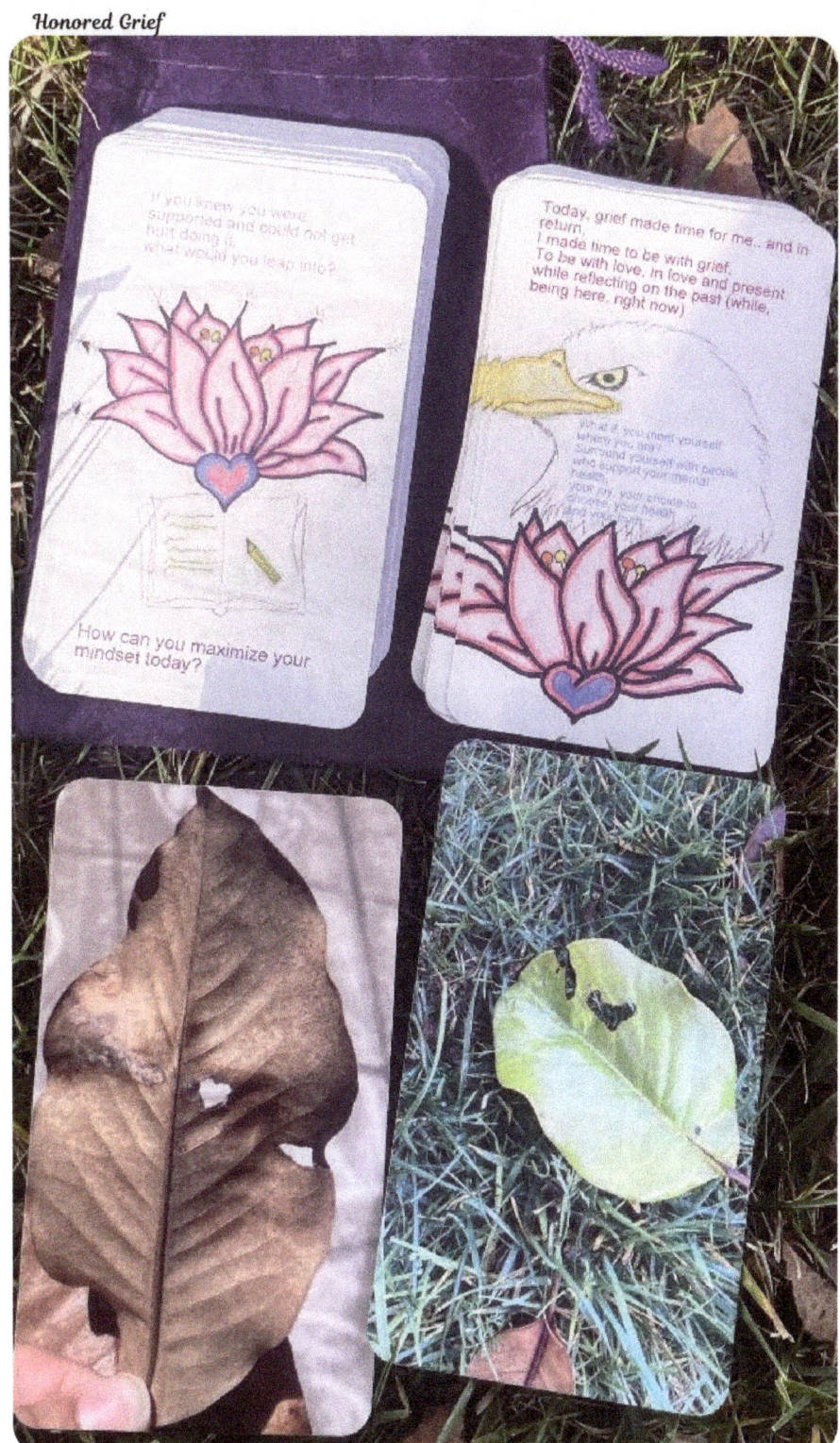

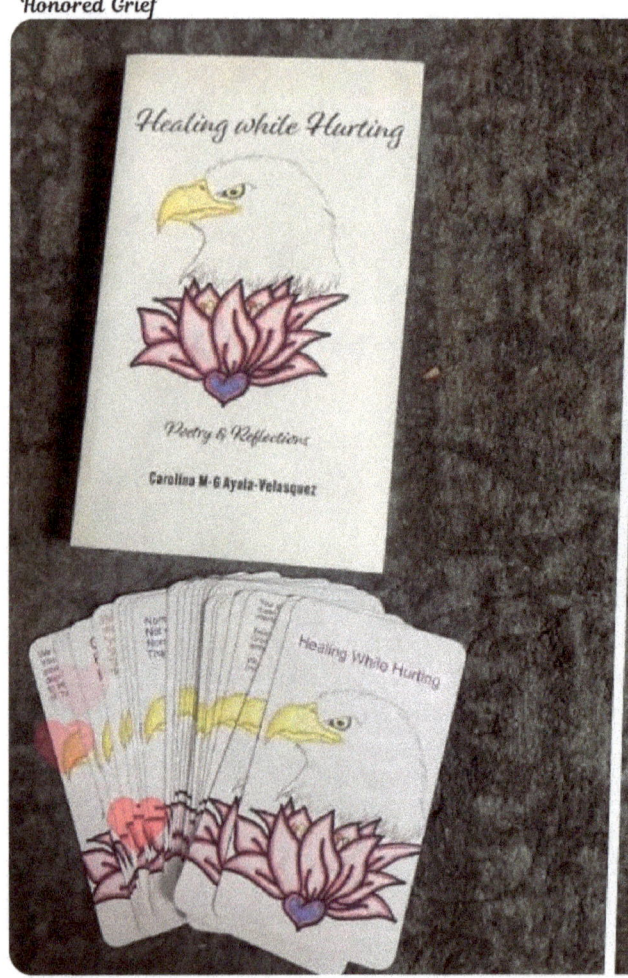

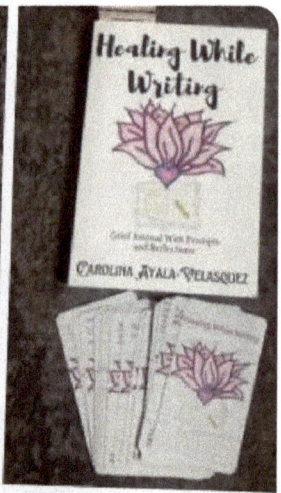

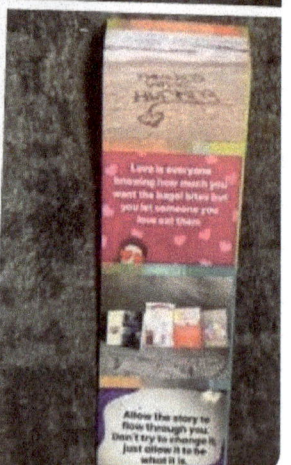

About The Author

Carolina Ayala (who many know as Lena) is a mother of 4 + griffin, their pandemic pup. She is a wife, a daughter and sister. She has taught infant/toddler care and pre-school formerly for about 7+years. She even taught child-development to high-schoolers and was a high school sub.

She is currently a health and wellness coach, a school crossing guard, a virtual assistant, and entrepreneur (authorship/workshops/pop up tables and speaking events.)

Thanks to the pandemic and the year before 2020, she started learning how to dream again and find herself outside of the titles of teacher and mother and wife. Pandemic times led back to childhood dreams that still were very real; dreams of becoming an author-finally. Honored grief is book number 8.

- Healing while hurting : poetry and reflections (published in 2020)
- Ratchet grandma: who's babysitting who (not for public sale) published in 2021
- Pandemic poetry and reflections (published in 2021)
- Gratitude saved me: journal prompts and reflections (published in 2022)
- Diary of a crossing guard: stargell and mosley (published in 2022)
- Healing while writing : grief journal with prompts and reflections (published in 2023)

- Cross guard chronicles: the diary continues (published in 2023)

She dreams of creating children's books, with her family as the artists. So, many books are in the "works." Including "Ratchet Grandma" the series.

This Book Was Beautifully Designed By Faith Alasonye Lotanna

If you'll love to have your book stunningly designed or you have any question concerning your book, you can Contact Me through:

Email:
falasonyelotanna@gmail.com

Mobile & Whatsapp Number:
+2348104323635

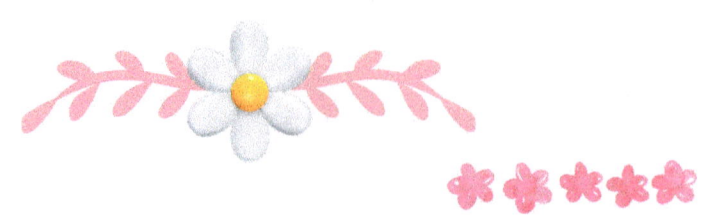